HARDCORE

ACKNOWLEDGMENTS

Art direction and design by Chris Hobrecker, with Lori Judd. Project Coordinator is Jeanine Detz.
Copyeditor is Maureen Meyers Farrar.
Photos by Robert Reiff, Chris Lund, Per Bernal, Ralph DeHaan, Alex Ardenti, Bob Gardner and Rick Schaff.

Chairman, President and CEO of AMI and Weider Publications, LLC is David Pecker.
Founding chairman is Joe Weider.
Group Editorial Director of *FLEX, MUSCLE & FITNESS* and *MUSCLE & FITNESS HERS* is Peter McGough.
Editor of *FLEX* is Michael Berg.

Published in 2007 by Triumph Books, 542 South Dearborn Street, Suite 750, Chicago, IL 60605.

Cover photos courtesy of Per Bernal.

ISBN 978-1-57243-973-3

Printed in China.

Some material contained herein previously published in *Flex* and *Muscle & Fitness* magazines.

HARDCORE

RONNIE COLEMAN'S
Complete Guide to
Weight Training

Ronnie Coleman, *IFBB pro, Mr. Olympia champion 1998–2005*
Edited by Michael Berg, NSCA-CPT

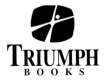

TRIUMPH
BOOKS

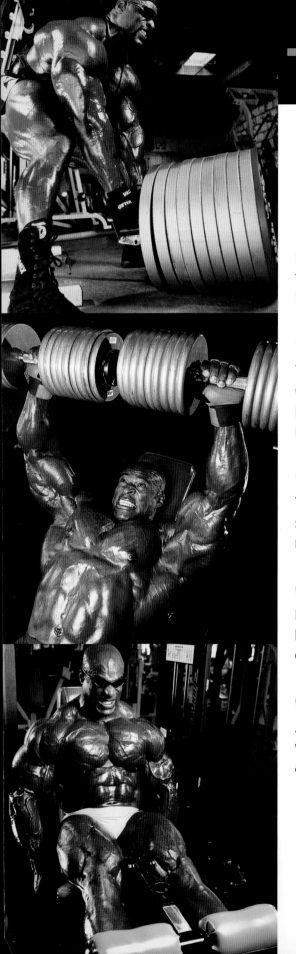

TABLE OF CONTENTS

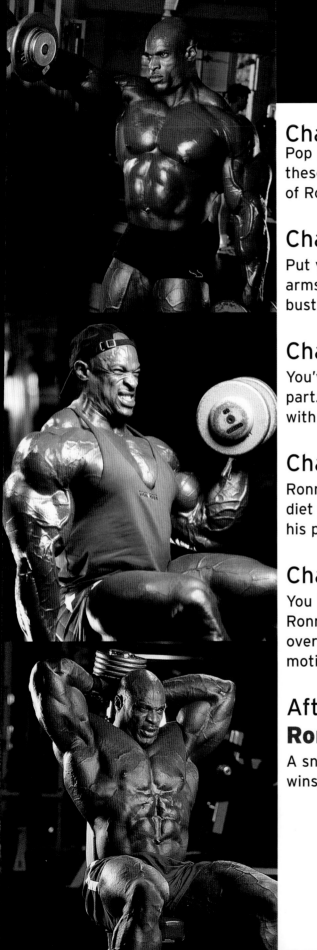

KING
OF THE MOUNTAIN

Chicago Pro Invitational, 11th. Night of Champions, 14th. Mr. Olympia, did not place.

Doesn't sound like a great opening salvo if you're a bodybuilder. But those results represent Ronnie Coleman's first year as a pro. That was 1992. In 1993 and 1994, his prospects started looking up, as he finished no lower than sixth in seven contests. In 1994, he even placed at the Mr. Olympia — it was only 15th, but it was progress.

In 1995, he won his first pro show, the Canada Pro Cup, a title he repeated a year later. At the 1995 Olympia, he climbed a few rungs again, to 11th, then he hit paydirt in '96 as he cracked the top six. Surely, steadily, he was making a name for himself.

But 1997 brought a setback, in the form of a ninth place finish at his fifth Mr. Olympia. His advancement up the ranks arrested in a doubt-inducing stumble, little did he know he was at a life-altering crossroads. Left to wonder just what it would take to change his fortunes and win the Olympia title, he found himself in a position where others may have been beaten down, their spirit crushed.

However, something else entirely happened with Coleman. He went back to his home in Texas, and set up shop once again in his favorite hardcore gym, MetroFlex. There, he honed and crafted what was already an elite-level physique into one that would shock the bodybuilding world and eventually shake it to its very foundations.

Flash forward one year. Reigning champion Dorian Yates retired, leaving the race for the Sandow trophy wide open. On stage at The Theater in Madison Square Garden in New York City, the drama unfolded, no one expecting the outcome or the aftermath. At that point, the very idea that the winner of that show would go on to tie the all-time record of eight Mr. Olympia victories by the great Lee Haney would have been deemed crazy.

Yet, it happened. Ronnie Coleman did the unthinkable that October night in 1998, jumping from ninth to first, snatching the title from precontest favorite Flex Wheeler, and setting a streak in motion that continued all the way through 2005.

Not bad from a man of humble beginnings. Born May 13, 1964, in Monroe, Louisiana, and reared in nearby Bastrop, Coleman was a big, strong kid from the time he was 12. He played on the football and baseball teams and ran track in school.

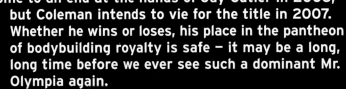

While he began training with weights in eighth grade, he wasn't pushed toward bodybuilding right away. In fact, playing football under legendary coach Eddie Robinson at Grambling State University, he was steered away from the heavy iron. "Robinson didn't believe in weight training," Coleman recalls. "He pretty much kept the same philosophy his whole career. He didn't even change the plays – he still ran the same ones from 1942!"

Coleman graduated with a degree in accounting, but after landing a job in that field, he decided he needed something more stimulating as a career. "In college, accounting was challenging, but at work it was the same thing over and over," he says. "So after two years, I quit and joined the Arlington, Texas police force, where I could use my mind as well as my body. One of the other officers talked me into going to the gym, and the owner, Brian Dobson, immediately offered me a free membership if I agreed to compete."

That gym was MetroFlex, and that handshake deal was struck in January 1990. Three short months passed and Coleman was vying for the Mr. Texas bodybuilding title, winning the heavyweight class and the overall honors. A year later, he earned his IFBB pro card at the World Amateur Championships, and his dual career of police officer and professional bodybuilder was born.

Arlington is a 100-square-mile incorporated area between Dallas and Fort Worth. For more than 10 years, Coleman patrolled the streets at least five shifts a week; the fact he was able to compete at the highest levels of pro bodybuilding during this time was an incredible feat of perseverance and discipline. When asked, though, he swears it wasn't that big of a deal. "I worked the afternoon shift, so I did my training early in the day and did my cardio after work, drank a protein shake and went to bed. The only problem I had is that I wasn't guaranteed a lunch break on the job, so finding time to eat when I needed to was difficult sometimes. I'd be riding down the street in a patrol car eating chicken and yams, but hey, you gotta do what you gotta do. It's just a matter of deciding what you want to do and then doing it. It's not that complicated. You just take care of business. You don't achieve anything worthwhile by making excuses and complaining about how hard it is."

Now retired from full-time police work, Coleman has worked diligently as the world's top bodybuilder, as he's traveled the world as an ambassador for the sport while putting in the hard efforts in the gym. As of this writing, his Olympia winning streak has come to an end at the hands of Jay Cutler in 2006,

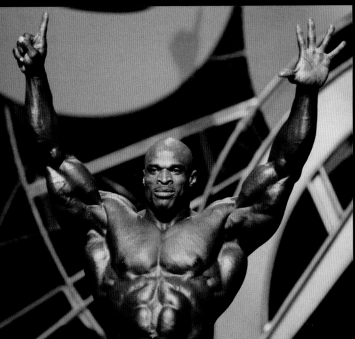

but Coleman intends to vie for the title in 2007. Whether he wins or loses, his place in the pantheon of bodybuilding royalty is safe – it may be a long, long time before we ever see such a dominant Mr. Olympia again.

A champion who has won against the odds, who has come back stronger than ever when almost everyone has counted him out, who has proven that hard work can earn you everything you've ever dreamed of. That's the Coleman legacy. With this book, you'll find a complete blueprint of how he did it; use it wisely, and you can blaze your own personal road to triumph.

– *Michael Berg, March 1, 2007*

CHAPTER 1

TRAINING PHILOSOPHY

My training philosophy can really be summed up in two words: Heavy and intense.

Of course, there is more to it than that, but it's the foundation on which everything else is built upon. I go to the gym six days a week, training every bodypart twice a week on average. I've been training the same way for years, and for one reason: It's worked. Six Sandow trophies on my mantle can't be wrong – I know my way around the gym, and in this book I want to share that knowledge with you.

A lot of people ask whether they should follow my rigid, demanding approach to training. From what I gather doing seminars meeting fans, I find many people can't follow my training split. Their bodies don't recover like mine does, so maybe they can work each bodypart only once a week. Others want to switch or adjust their training splits instinctively. That's fine. You must eventually find your own way, through trial and error, although I believe I provide a great blueprint to start you on your way. Here are some of my basic tenets, which provide the framework upon which the training in the rest of this book is based.

RULE 1
Free weights should make up the majority of your exercise selections. In my routine, I'd say free-weight moves constitute at least 75% of my training arsenal, with the rest of the exercises done with cables and machines. I'll use a machine when there's not a good barbell or dumbbell equivalent for a certain bodypart, such as calves, or if I'm just looking for a change of pace. But when it comes to the bread and butter of my training, the free-weight room is the location of choice.

RULE 2
Bilateral (two-limb) movements should be more prevalent in your routine than unilateral (one-limb-at-a-time) moves. I generally do the bulk of my exercises with two arms or legs at a time, with some exceptions, of course. Unilateral movements, such as concentration curls for biceps, have their place in a workout, but you build the base of your size and strength through compound moves, like barbell squats, barbell and dumbbell rows, deadlifts, flat and incline bench presses and seated and standing military presses. Some people like to do unilateral stuff to isolate one muscle if it's lagging its counterpart on the other side, but most of my bodyparts are pretty much equal.

RULE 3
Intensity is everything when it comes to making appreciable gains. While some of your sessions may be more intense than others, you should be focused, alert and giving your all every time you step into the weight room. Any less, and you may be simply spinning your wheels. Intensity is also a combination of poundage, speed, rest periods — any number of such variables can be manipulated to your advantage.

RULE 4
Continually strive to get stronger. The heavier you go, the more muscle you're going to build. But even when you go heavy, remember that you still have to get in your repetitions, too. As you'll see in the workouts outlined in this book, my philosophy is that if you aren't doing at least 10–15 reps per set, you aren't really building anything. I mostly do 10–15 reps; the only time I go below, say, eight reps is when I'm doing a strength-oriented move like deadlifts. I'll perform more than 15 on warm-up sets and for the working sets of an exercise like leg extensions. I always do a warm-up set before the working sets of every exercise.

RULE 5
Going to failure on your exercises isn't as important as going to full muscle fatigue in your workout. I'll explain this more in Chapter 10, but for now, know this: Going to muscle failure on a few sets in your workout won't give you gains over time like making sure you fully fatigue a muscle by doing at least 15 hard 'n' heavy sets in your workout for each major bodypart.

RULE 6
Variety is good; complete revolution is not. To quell boredom and to keep your muscles from adapting to the same exact routine, you should work different techniques and exercises into your workout each time you train, but you shouldn't radically change your philosophy day to day, week to week, or month to month — find something that works and stick to it long-term, making only minor adjustments. Doing low reps and heavy weights one week, then jumping to high reps and ridiculously light weights the next won't give you the gains you seek.

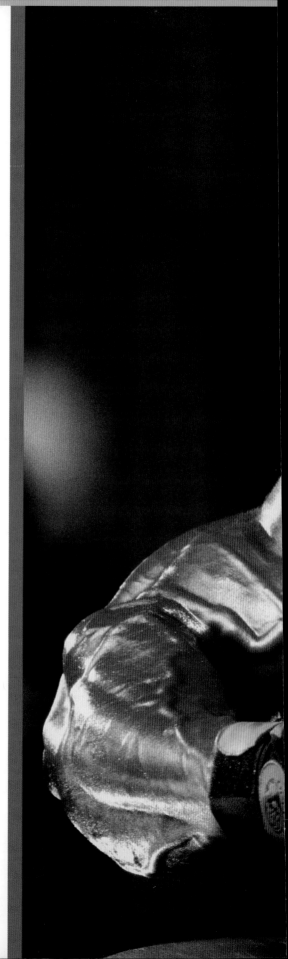

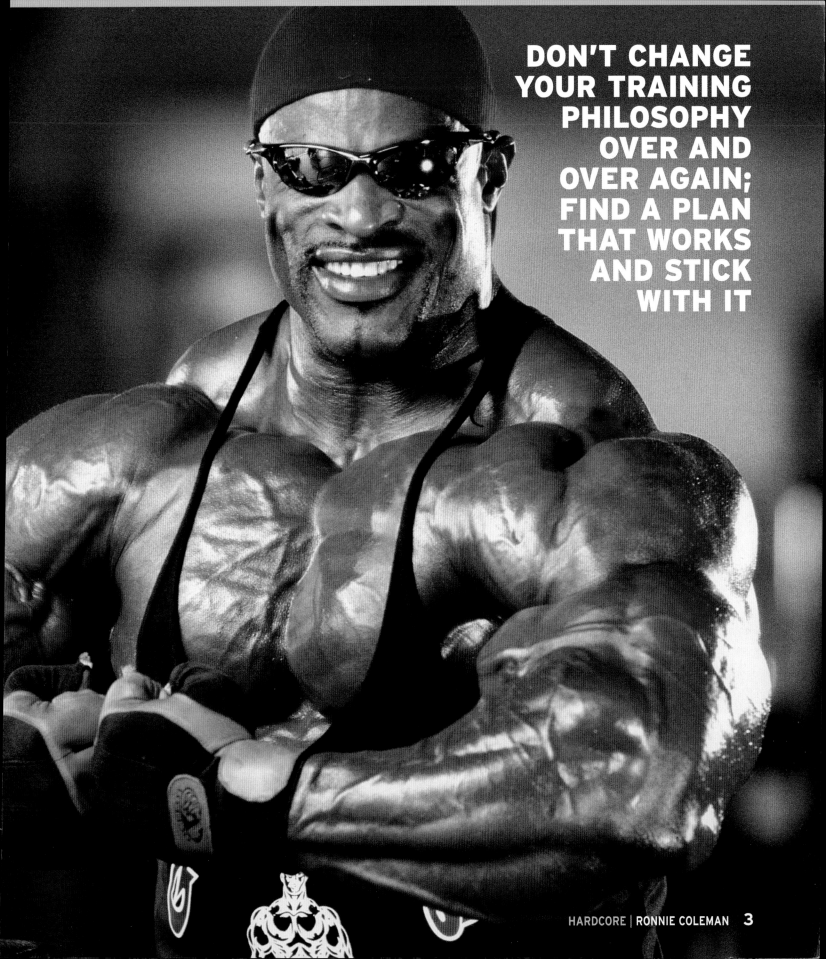

DON'T CHANGE YOUR TRAINING PHILOSOPHY OVER AND OVER AGAIN; FIND A PLAN THAT WORKS AND STICK WITH IT

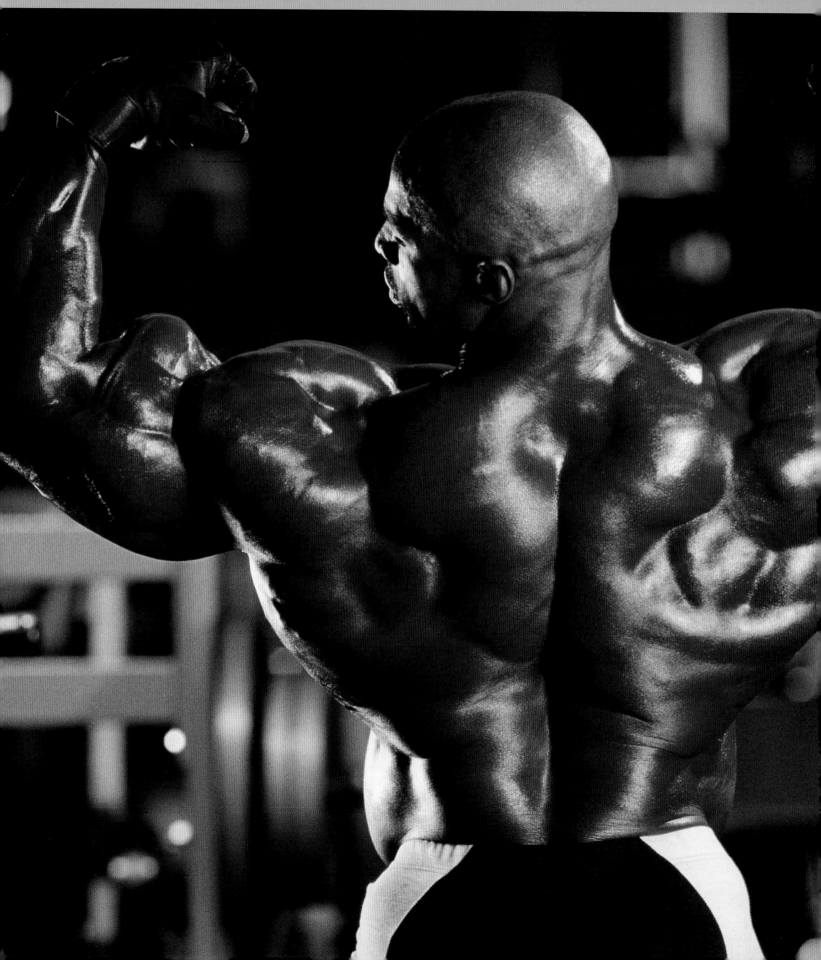

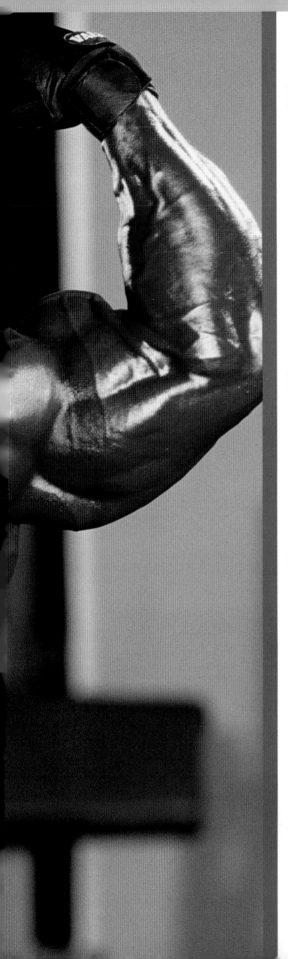

RULE 7 Be a stickler for exercise form on every set and every single repetition you do. Yes, usually there's more than one "right" way to perform an exercise. Having said that, there's definitely a wrong way, too. Do all your movements strictly, maintaining control over the weight at all times. There's a certain form of "cheating" that's okay in some instances (pushing through a sticking point), and on explosive movements you don't want to necessarily plod through the positive portion of a repetition. But for the most part, make perfect form a priority and you won't go wrong.

RULE 8 Drop the cardio from your training schedule when you want to get bigger, and pick it up when you want to cut up. I do very little cardio in my off-season, but I usually add regular cardio back in about 11 weeks out from a contest. I do it in the morning right before I work out and then again late at night, before I go to bed.

RULE 9 You've heard this before, but it's important: For the sake of your health and your muscle, you need to drink a lot of water. Keeping yourself hydrated during your workouts and throughout the day is key to sustaining your energy. Hard-training bodybuilders drink up to a gallon a day, but you can start with less — about 8–12 cups — and work upward from there.

RULE 10 When in doubt, eat clean, even in the off-season. Sure, you can get big on ice cream, potato chips, pizza — big and fat, that is. I've learned many tough lessons throughout my career, and now, instead of getting lackadaisical with my eating habits when not prepping for a contest, I keep my diet clean year-round. I go more into more depth on my own diet in Chapter 9, but the bottom line is, the cleaner your diet — foods such as fish, chicken breast, turkey breast, steak, vegetables, fruits, and whole grains — the better your results.

RULE 11 Use the tools of the trade to help you. I use devices such as chalk for grip strength, gloves, wrist straps, lifting belts — if it helps you lift more, it's all good.

RULE 12 Be consistent. This may be the most important rule of all, because sticking with your training and diet over the long haul can even help you overcome other mistakes you might make. A guy who doesn't have the perfect training program but doesn't miss workouts and meals will always come out on top vs. someone who has the perfect plan but constantly falls off the wagon. A lot of people fall into the habit of skipping workouts, but the key to long-term success is paying your dues, week after week, year upon year, decade into decade. Accept no excuses, because there are none.

Now, let's move on to the training — a bodypart-by-bodypart sample of how I've prepared for the Mr. Olympia contest over the years, starting with my favorite, and perhaps my most famous, bodypart in Chapter 2: Back.

CHAPTER 2
BUILD A BIGGER
BACK

In my opinion, two bodyparts represent the dividing line between the wanna-be's and the true, hardcore lifters: Back and legs. Developing either of these muscle groups take superhuman effort, unwavering concentration and pure will. You see a guy with impossibly full, barn-door-wide lats or redwood-thick legs, you know he takes his efforts at the gym very seriously.

I've been told my back is one of the best the sport has ever seen, and I take that as a great compliment. It makes the years of balls-to-the-wall deadlifts, fiber-ripping rows and lat-swelling pull-ups worthwhile.

To craft a showstopping back, there are no shortcuts – you have to pay your dues through sweat, pain and heavy, heavy weights. If you're ready to make that commitment, keep reading.

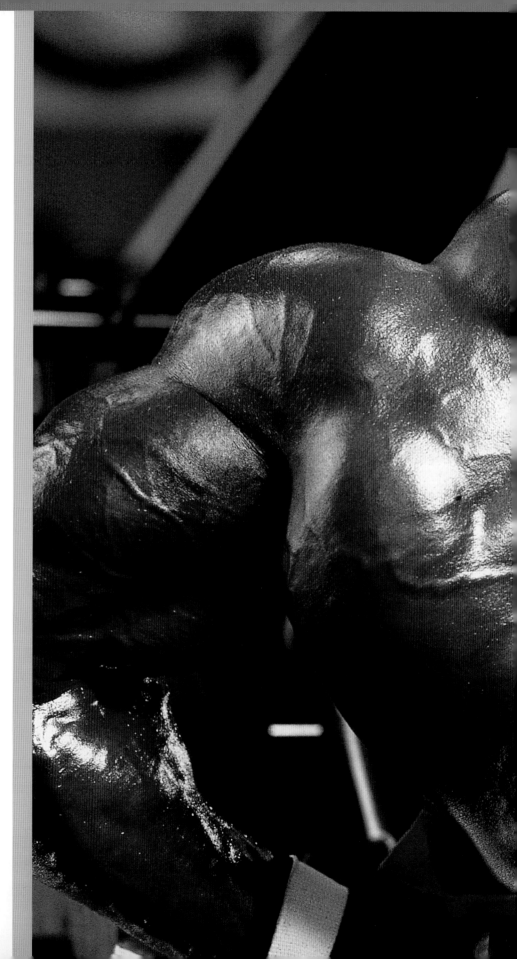

BACK DAY BEGINS with T-bar rows, first with a light set to warm up followed by three heavy sets. I pyramid up, but against "conventional" bodybuilding wisdom, I don't drop my reps as the poundage increases. I keep going for 12, reaching down deep inside to power through the final excruciating reps. High reps, heavy weight — in that regard, my training philosophy hasn't changed much since I began lifting.

Next, I continue with an exercise that isolates each side of my back: one-arm dumbbell rows. When I perform these reps I do go semi-slow — never super-slow — controlling that dumbbell instead of just hoisting it full speed to my flank. But because I'm going to the dusty, not-so-popular end of the dumbbell rack, I don't hold those monsters up in the top position for a long squeeze. I lift, I contract hard, I return to the start. Strive for that same steady pace in your sets.

After I hit the rows, I switch gears to pull-ups and pulldowns. Rows build the mountains of thickness; pulls widen your lats. When you do the pull-up, if you find you're not strong enough to do a 12-rep set, work your way up to it. Arnold had a great trick for doing just that. Take the amount of reps you want to complete — if you follow the routine I provide, that would be 36 — and proceed to do as many sets as it takes to hit that number. That could be three sets of 10, one set of six. Or four sets of eight, one set of four . . . you get the idea. Stick to that program, and you will get strong enough to knock out 3 sets of 12 in a month or two.

Pulldowns may be the last exercise of the day, but that doesn't mean it's time to hit cruise control. Take pulldowns as seriously as you do your first exercise — challenge yourself on your weight selection, and don't rock backwards on each repetition to get the bar down to your chest. Pull with your back, elbows out, chest lifted and lower back tight and arched. Be the guy they call "Textbook" in the gym.

RONNIE'S BACK WORKOUT

EXERCISE	SETS	REPS
T-Bar Row (warm-up)	1	15
(working sets)	3	12
One-Arm Dumbbell Row	3-4	12
Wide-Grip Pull-Up	3	12
Front Pulldown	3-4	12

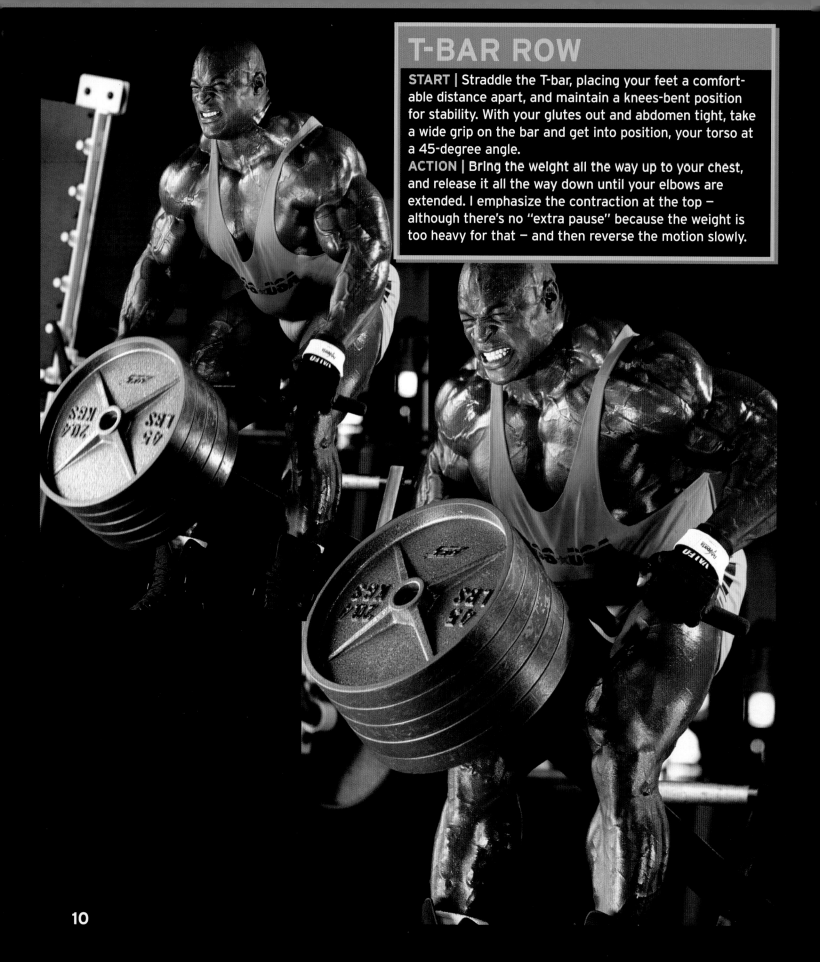

T-BAR ROW

START | Straddle the T-bar, placing your feet a comfortable distance apart, and maintain a knees-bent position for stability. With your glutes out and abdomen tight, take a wide grip on the bar and get into position, your torso at a 45-degree angle.

ACTION | Bring the weight all the way up to your chest, and release it all the way down until your elbows are extended. I emphasize the contraction at the top — although there's no "extra pause" because the weight is too heavy for that — and then reverse the motion slowly.

ONE-ARM DUMBBELL ROW

START | Place one leg on a flat bench, one foot on the floor for stability. Lean forward from the hips, holding your abs tight to protect your spine.

ACTION | Bring the weight all the way up to your chest, your elbow moving up toward the ceiling, and then lower the weight all the way down toward the floor. Allow the weight to move straight down, stretching out your lats but maintaining a slight bend in your elbow in the bottom position. Repeat the movement for reps. Vary the position of the dumbbell occasionally, from (a) keeping it parallel to the body throughout, to (b) beginning palm-backward at the bottom and supinating as you pull.

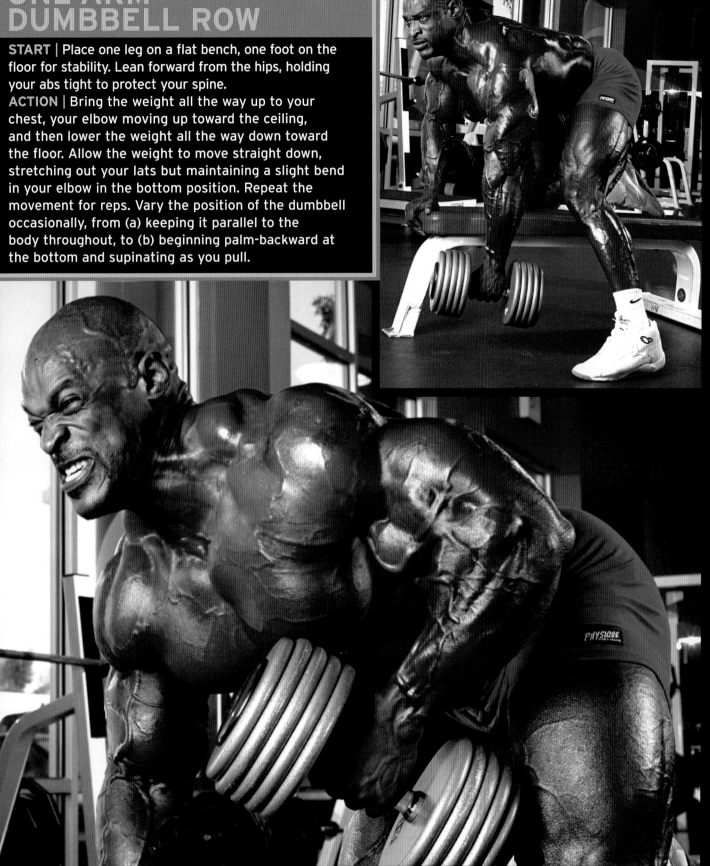

WIDE-GRIP PULL-UP

START | I like the way this exercise pumps my lats, so it's a staple in my back workouts throughout the year, whether off-season or deep in contest preparation. It's so valuable that I'd call it the No. 1 back exercise, especially for a beginner or intermediate. You simply can't build a complete back without it. The pull-up also provides a good gauge of your own strength (which is likely why the military uses it), because it's a direct measure of your pulling power to your bodyweight — if you're so heavy that you can't do a pull-up effectively, I'd argue you're probably carrying a lot more fat than muscle. To begin, you'll jump up and take a wide grip on the bar — I go out as far as the bar will let me go, although a grip just outside shoulder width will do if you prefer. Drop your body completely into a dead hang position, arms straight and feet off the floor (you can either cross them, as shown here, or simply bend your knees).

ACTION | Contract your lats hard as you pull yourself upward. Often people make the mistake of not giving enough effort in this move — you really need to psych yourself up for a big-time pull, just as though you were about to do a heavy deadlift. After all, you're moving a lot of weight straight up against gravity. This definitely requires more power than a finesse exercise. On the ascent, I try to rise all the way up and put my chin over the bar. Then I lower myself slowly, keeping my elbows slightly bent (to protect the tendons in the elbow from hyperextending) as I reach the bottom dead-hang position again. Throughout the exercise, keep your elbows flared out; the more they come in to your sides, the bigger part of the load your biceps take on.

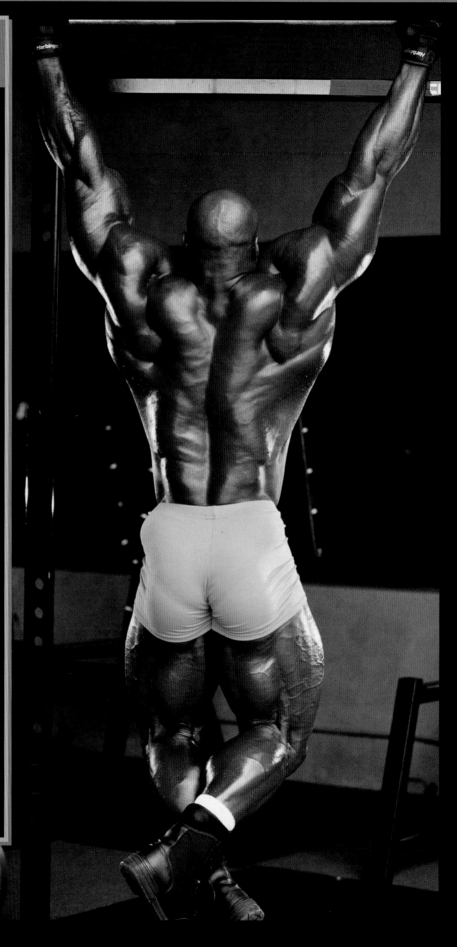

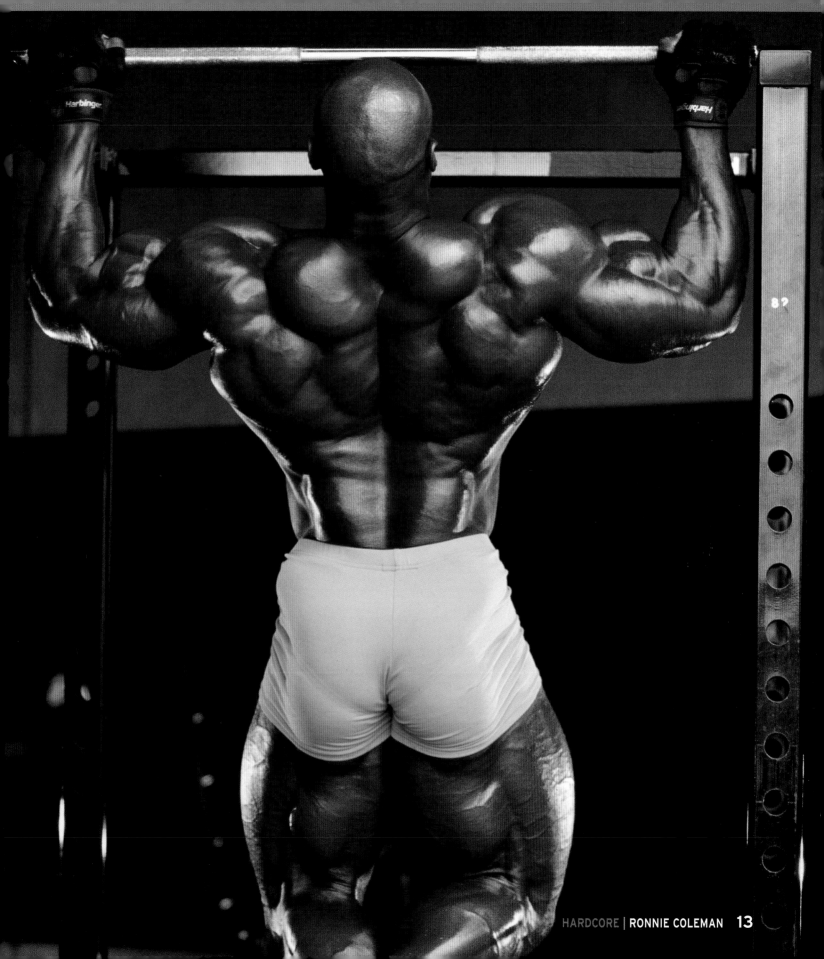

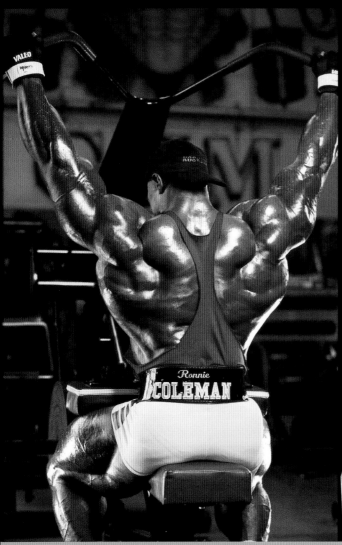

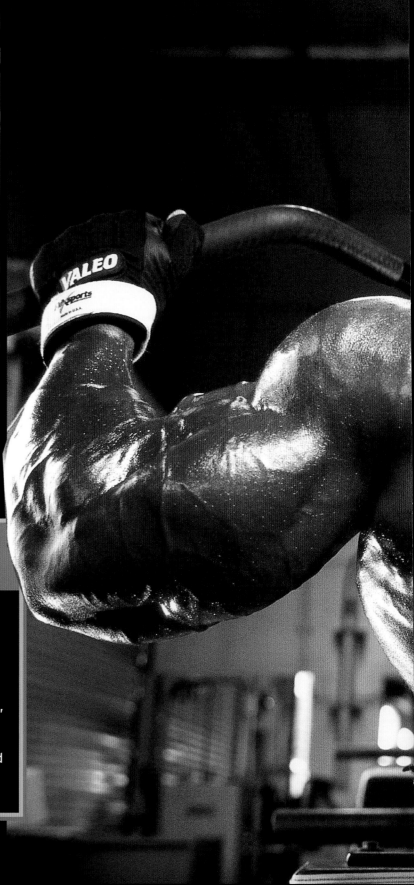

PULLDOWN TO FRONT

START | Position yourself at the pulldown machine, adjusting the seat so that your knees fit snugly under the pads with your feet firmly planted on the floor. Take a wide grip on the bar.

ACTION | I tilt back just a little bit and focus on using my lat strength – not my biceps – to bring the bar down all the way to my chest. I get a good contraction, then release the weight back up. With the heavy weight I use, I'm careful to keep good form and maintain control through the entire movement. I get a good stretch through my lats at the top of the movement, and keep my elbows slightly bent to protect the joint.

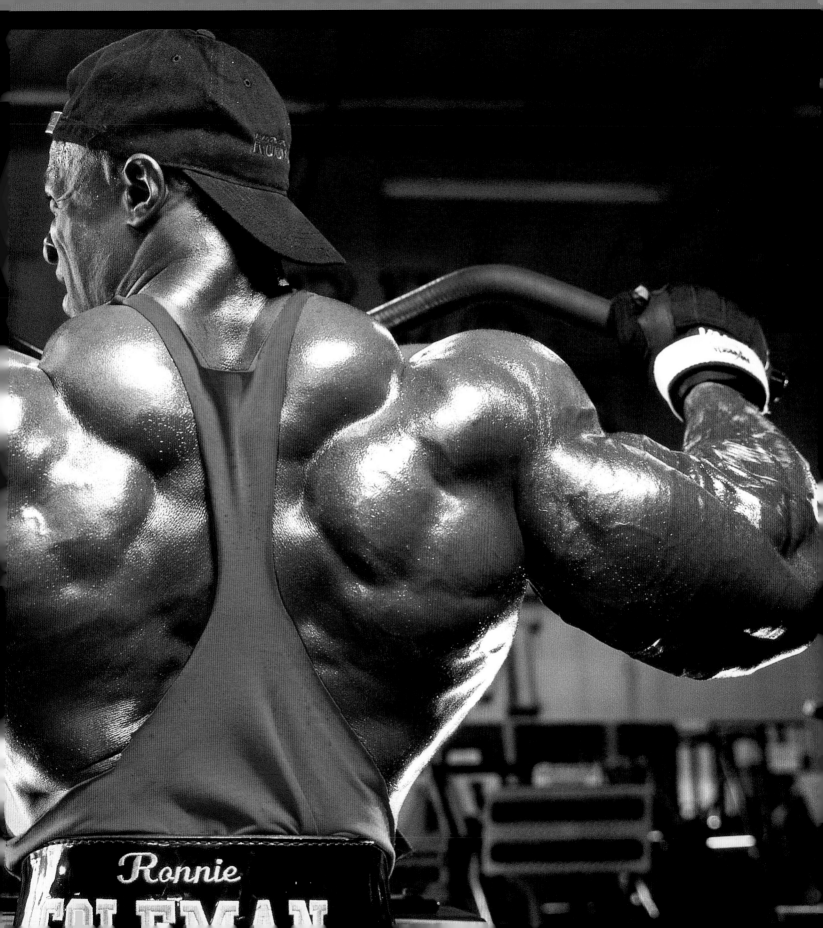

Final Notes

The routine I provide here has served me well many, many times, but it doesn't represent the one and only back regimen I ever do. You need some variety, not only to keep your workouts interesting, but also to brutalize your back in a multitude of ways. If you feed it the same exercises all the time, your back will adjust — and stop responding.

I cycle in different exercises, and you should, too. Changing it up stimulates growth and helps you consistently improve over time. Deadlifts, barbell rows and Hammer-Strength pulldowns are some of the many great choices. Starting on this page, I highlight some of my favorite alternates. Switch some of these in and out of your workout, making sure to keep an equal balance of rows and pulldowns/pull-ups.

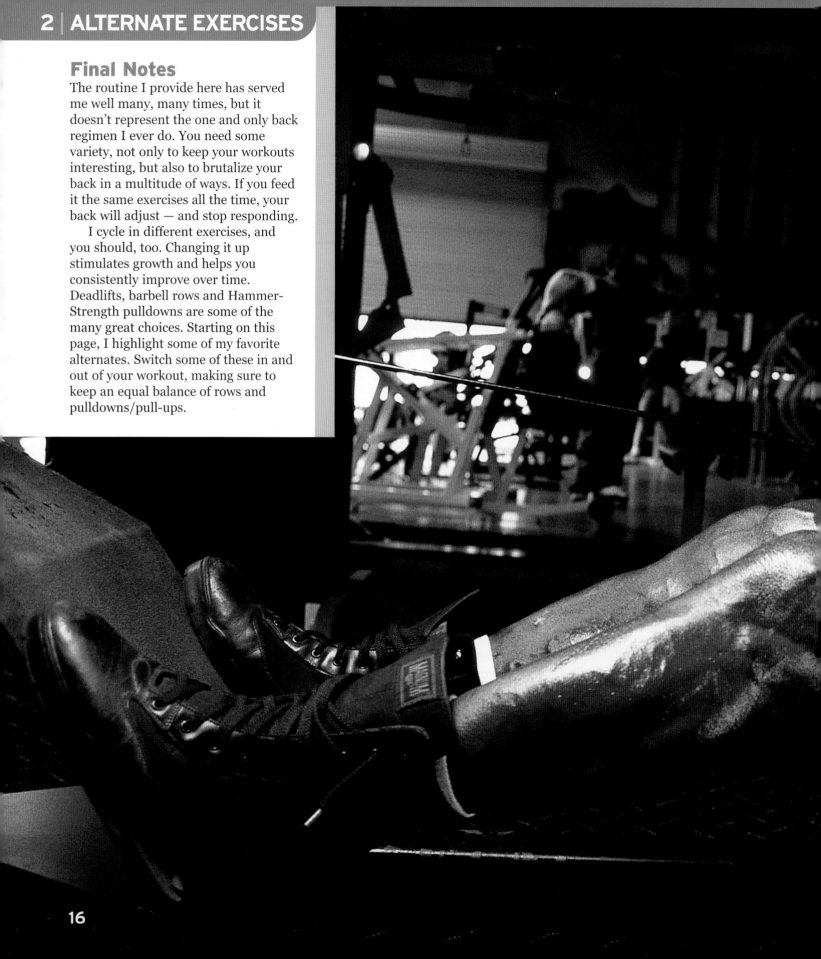

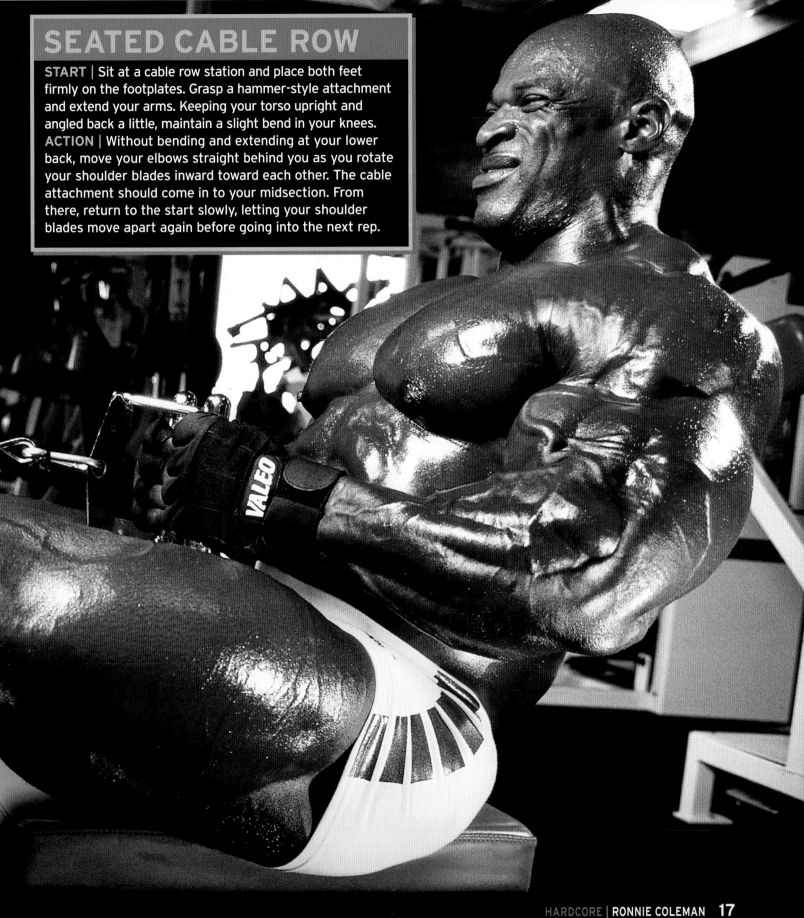

SEATED CABLE ROW

START | Sit at a cable row station and place both feet firmly on the footplates. Grasp a hammer-style attachment and extend your arms. Keeping your torso upright and angled back a little, maintain a slight bend in your knees.

ACTION | Without bending and extending at your lower back, move your elbows straight behind you as you rotate your shoulder blades inward toward each other. The cable attachment should come in to your midsection. From there, return to the start slowly, letting your shoulder blades move apart again before going into the next rep.

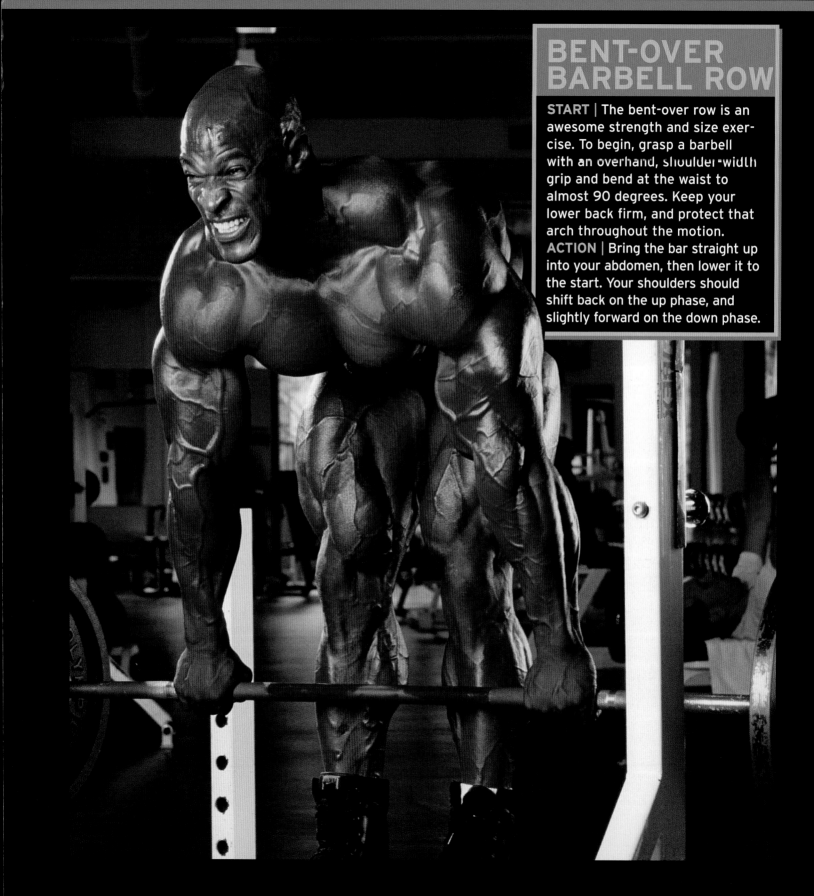

BENT-OVER BARBELL ROW

START | The bent-over row is an awesome strength and size exercise. To begin, grasp a barbell with an overhand, shoulder-width grip and bend at the waist to almost 90 degrees. Keep your lower back firm, and protect that arch throughout the motion.
ACTION | Bring the bar straight up into your abdomen, then lower it to the start. Your shoulders should shift back on the up phase, and slightly forward on the down phase.

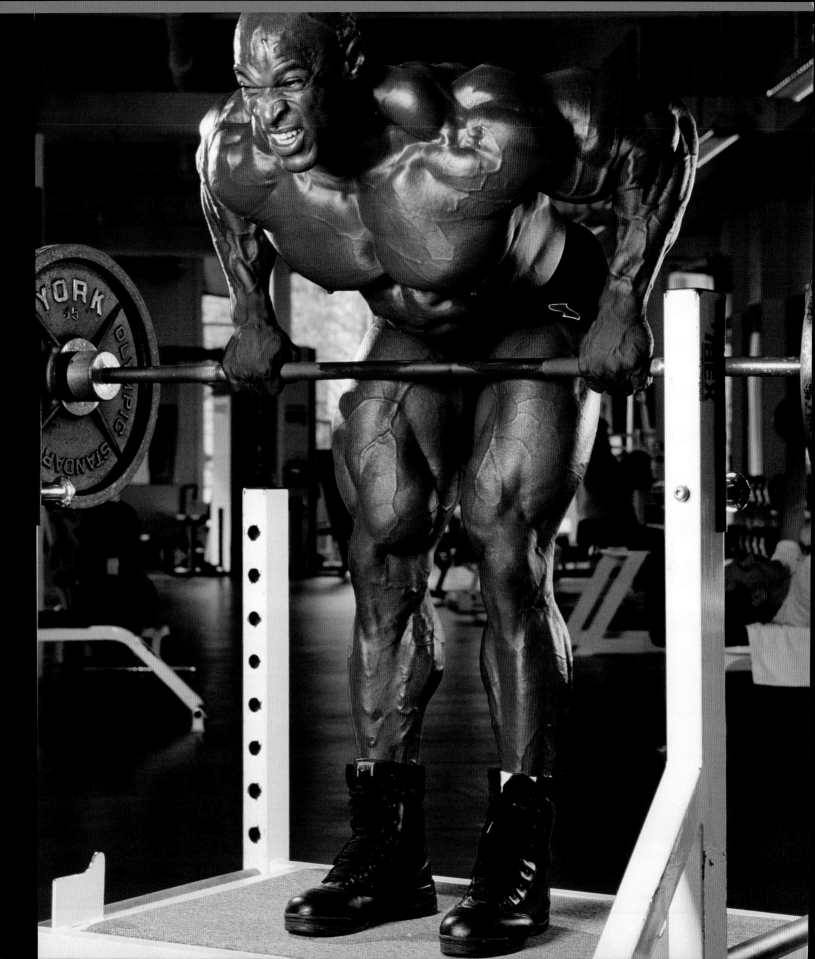

Ronnie's Lat Lessons

1 USE STANDING COMPOUND EXERCISES in all your bodypart routines. Your back is the structure on which the rest of your body hangs. As a result, it will share in the weight-training benefits of other bodyparts, if it shares in the exercise for that other bodypart. My parking-lot lunges are a good example. For those, I lunge back and forth across the parking lot of my gym with a 225-pound barbell on my back. Although that is a legs-day exercise, you can imagine what it does for my traps and my entire back, including my upper lats, rhomboids and the full length of my erectors. It's also a terrific strength-builder, and the greater my back strength, the more weight I can lift for more reps, resulting in faster growth. Other free-standing exercises that enhance the muscularity of your back are squats, barbell curls, standing overhead french presses, upright rows, military presses and front barbell or dumbbell raises. Of course, the more weight you use for those, the harder your back has to work.

2 DEADLIFT. From the first time I grabbed a barbell in my early teens, through the days I was a competitive powerlifter in high school, to now as the number one bodybuilder in the world, deadlifts have been an anchor exercise of my back work-outs. I have always done them. Deadlifts are the only exercise that require the combined strength of every muscle in your back, thereby distributing size and thickness over the entire area in the most natural and perfect proportions. From

beginning to end, the deadlift movement hits everything, at one point or another. The initial lift at the bottom thickens your erectors and pulls your lats low into your sides, the middle arc widens and thickens your barn doors, and the lockout at the top turns you into Quasimodo. It's shown from the midpoint at left.

Start with the bar on the floor, take a shoulder-width overhand grip on the bar, bend deep at your knees, and tense your entire body. Keeping your lower back arched throughout, drive through your heels to lift the bar along your legs until you reach a standing position. Lower back down the same path until the weights touch down, then go into the next repetition.

3 ROW. By rows, I mean any rowing motion in which you stretch your arms to the front and pull into your mid-section, the purpose being to widen the two slabs of meat that compose the latissimus dorsi and to bring out muscular detail in the middle and upper back. My favorites are barbell rows, T-bar rows and seated pulley rows. Each provides the same general development, as well as unique benefits. Barbell rows are for lat width and mass, erector thickness, middle- and upper-back muscularity, and for adding mass to the lower trapezius. T-bar rows are also for lat width and mass, with emphasis on middle- and upper-back muscularity. Seated pulley rows lower the sweep of your lats and bring out striations along both sides of your erectors. I use one or two of these in every back workout. All

three offer varying degrees of mass-vs.-isolation benefits: barbell rows for the most mass, seated pulley rows for the most isolation, and T-bar rows for the best combination of both.

4 PULL FROM OVERHEAD. Deads and rows will give you all the width and thickness you need, but the only way to bring out the density and separations of the teres, infraspinatus, rhomboid and lower trapezius muscles in the upper-middle back is by pulling from overhead. Where lifts and rows move the lats from front to back, overhead pulls rotate the lats downward and inward against each other through the same plane, as if they are two grinding wheels edge to edge, crushing all of those minor back muscles between them. The best exercises for this motion are machine pulldowns, cable pulldowns and wide-grip chins or pull-ups. To emphasize the width of your upper lats and the muscularity of your middle back, use front pulldowns or pull-ups. To thicken the lower triangle of your traps and separate your rhomboids, teres and spinatus muscles, pull as low as you can behind your neck.

5 FIND THE POINT OF TRUE FAILURE. I've never believed in going to failure, because a weak-willed sub-conscious will always find a way to "fail" too early. Here's what I do to keep myself from wimping out: I use, as my goal for the set, the maximum number of reps I've ever been able to attain with that

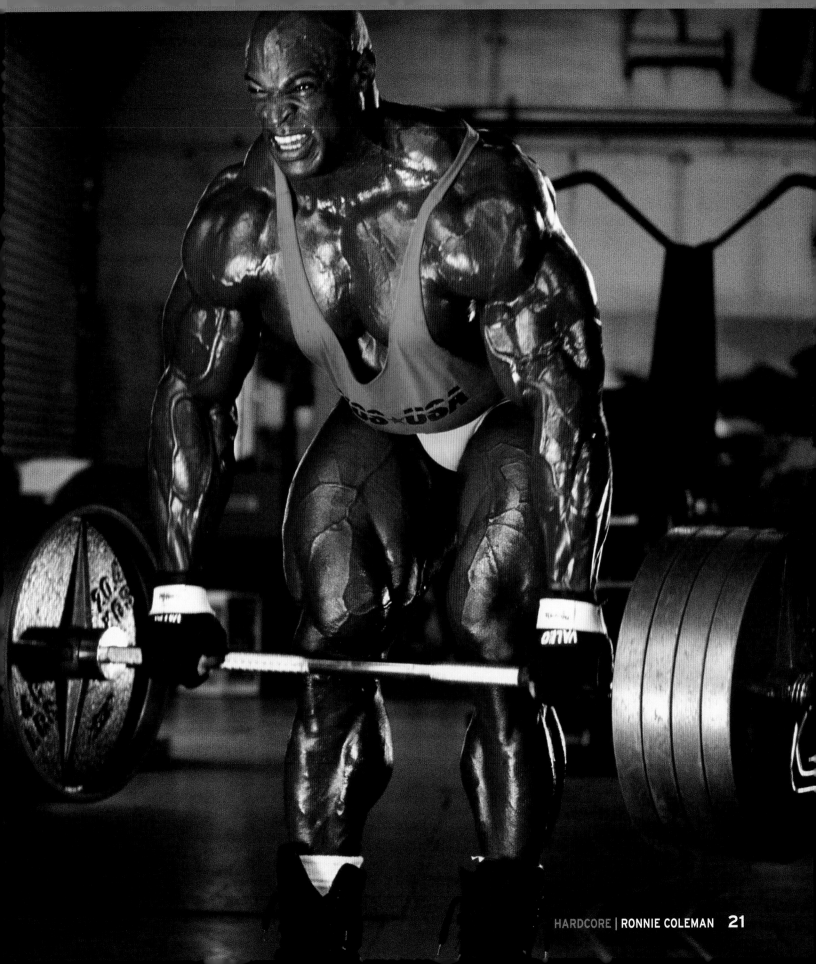

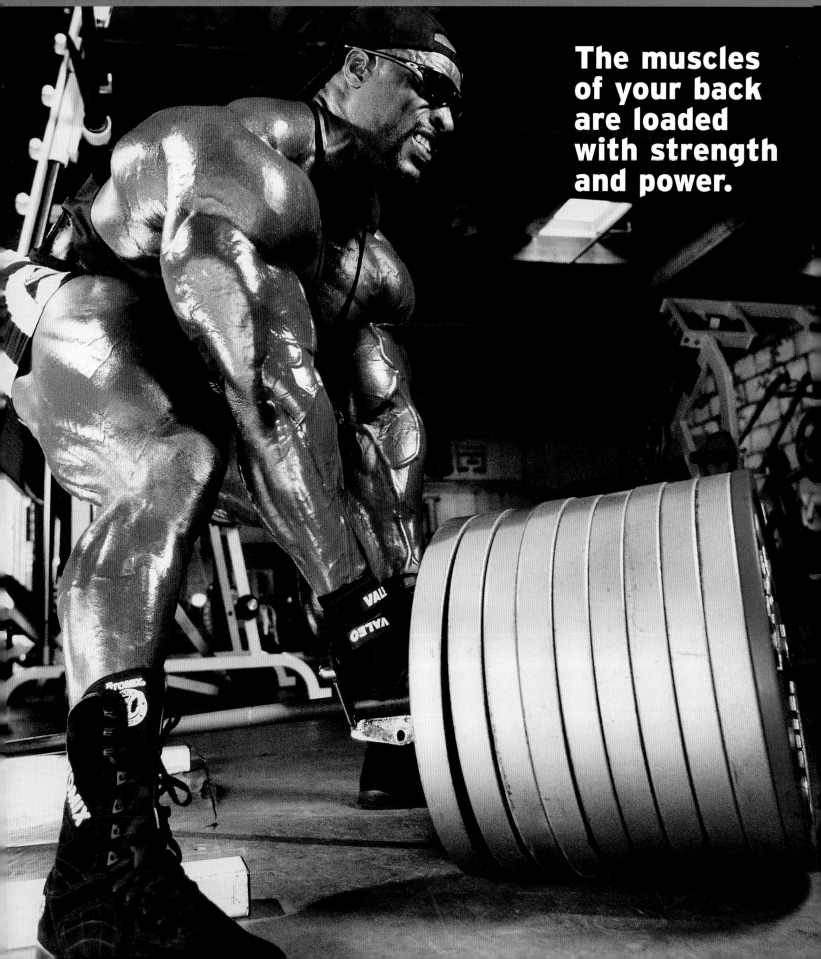

The muscles of your back are loaded with strength and power.

weight. My first commitment, then, is to make sure I do not fail until I've done at least that many repetitions. However, I have a second commitment: namely, to try to push past my failure number. It's a mind game I play on my body, and it forces me to constantly strive to raise my level of training and development. Eventually, I can do more reps in a certain exercise and then I adjust the weight upward. I have yet to find a better motivational tool. Not only do I hit an intensity high as I reach my numerical goal, but when I pass it, my self-esteem soars to a new high as well. At that point, I feel as though I'm Superman. More important, I've worked the muscle harder than I ever thought I could, and I can then rest in the knowledge that my growth will be more than I had hoped.

6 GO HEAVY . . . AND I MEAN REALLY HEAVY.

A great back is one that has the landscape of an Arizona prison rock pile, with fissures and peaks so jagged that they'd rip out the undercarriage of my Hummer if I happened to run over the guy. That kind of back doesn't come from "surgical-precision" bodybuilding, in which you work each muscle separately by means of tiny twitchy contractions. Your back is too complex for that. One muscle works the next, and so on. Ideally, you should work your back in areas, rather than aim for individual muscles, and only heavy weight can force you to do that. Also, instead of pressing, as is the case with exercises for other muscle groups, your back muscles lift like a crane, which means your back has almost double the strength over other bodyparts. Train it as such by doubling the weight. Since you're pulling, you'll also find that the greater your range of motion, the greater your strength, so doubling the weight doubles the benefits of a full movement, as well.

7 DON'T CHEAT YOURSELF out of a full range of motion.

Since your back doesn't have any levered joints, its muscles can only be thoroughly stressed by allowing your arms and shoulders to stretch them through their maximum range of motion. With other bodyparts, such as arms and legs, you'll know when you're getting a full range of motion by the pump or burn that develops in the muscle belly, but a full range of motion with your back is indicated only by a hard pull at the muscle insertions. For every extension, maintain tension, and let the weight stretch your lats and shoulders as deep as possible. As you contract, pull back with your shoulders as you stick out your chest and try to scissor your lats together behind you. For your initial, higher-rep sets, use the peak contraction principle: Get an extra-hard one-second squeeze with all of the muscles in the area before beginning your next extension. With deadlifts, locking out your shoulders at the top is your peak contraction.

8 KEEP CHANGE A CONSTANT in your workout.

Because of your back's complexity and size, it needs to be hit with every conceivable combination of stresses, to make sure no muscle is ever neglected. No consecutive workouts should ever be exactly the same. Even if I use the same exercises, at least some other variable will change. This doesn't mean I don't have favorites. Quite the contrary: deadlifts, pull-ups, bent-over barbell rows, T-bar rows, seated pulley rows and pulldowns are stalwarts in my workouts. Many other exercises are rarities, but I do get around to them eventually.

9 NEVER LET UP. In my mind, there's absolutely no such thing as "precontest training"

and no such thing as a light day. Every workout, every exercise – whether a compound or isolation move – gets my full impassioned fury, and I never do less in a workout than I did in the one that preceded it. Right up to a show, I'm trying to increase my weights and my reps. As I mentioned earlier, I may do a single with 800 pounds for deadlifts in one workout, but that doesn't mean I won't work just as hard for 12 reps of seated cable rows in the next workout. Believe in the dictum that every rep, if performed to the maximum of your capability, builds muscle, and the more resistance you're fighting against during that rep, the more muscle it builds. When your progress seems to come to a screeching stop, that's the time to say to the weight, "See you on the other side, brother" – then throw on more plates and set a new record for your lift, just for spite. In the world of human performance and potential, the body usually exceeds the realm of expectation; my guess is you'll usually find you're stronger than you ever give yourself credit for.

CHAPTER 3

A CHAMPIONSHIP
CHEST

Admit it . . . some of you out there cracked open this book and went straight for this chapter. Yep, for some, there's chest and then there's "all the other bodyparts."

Of course, this is where you'd expect me to say, that's not a good attitude — that you shouldn't short-shrift the rest of your body while going all out on your pecs. It's true, you shouldn't, but just the same, I can't blame you either.

No doubt about it, chest day is fun. I love the powerful feeling you get out of pressin' heavy tonnage. I love the fact that you can really pump out your pectorals, each rep pouring more blood into the muscles until they're bulging against your skin. And when you look in the mirror, they're right in your face; instant gratification for the hard work you're putting in.

I don't condone working your chest at the expense of your other training — in fact, you should instead try to get the same feeling for all your bodyparts — but man, I totally understand where you're coming from.

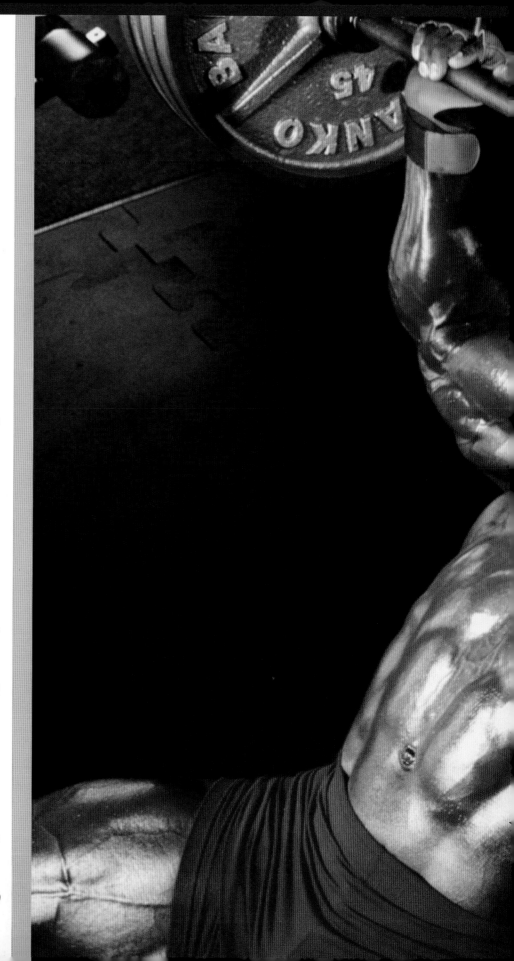

EVERYTHING I'VE ACCOMPLISHED IN BODYBUILDING can be traced back to my days as a competitive powerlifter in Bastrop, Louisiana. It may sound strange, but the seeds of my bodybuilding career were sown during long afternoons of bench pressing, squatting and deadlifting for the Bastrop High School powerlifting team.

Bastrop, a small town outside of Monroe in northeast Louisiana, was the sort of town where football is king. I was a pretty good football player in junior high school; in fact, I garnered a reputation for being particularly strong and powerful.

Once word spread, the powerlifters in high school decided to recruit me for some down-in-the-trenches lifting and competition. Derrick Harris, a fellow powerlifter from my hometown, was the lightning rod who got me going. With a steady diet of the meat-and-potatoes exercise, I built heaps of power and laid the foundation for the muscle maturity I possess today.

That heavy-lifting mindset is still there, but now the brute force of those early workouts is coupled with bodybuilding tenets for better overall development. For instance, the two training programs in this chapter illustrate what I did to prepare my chest for my second Mr. Olympia title in 1999. The All-Barbell Workout includes flat, incline and decline presses, finishing with machine flyes. The All-Dumbbell Workout also includes the three types of presses, ending with incline flyes.

I try to hit my chest twice per week. For instance, if I do the all-barbell workout on Wednesday, I'll come back to the gym on Saturday for the all-dumbbell attack.

I perform one warm-up set of 15–20 light reps on the first chest exercise of the day. After that, my pecs are pumped, bursting with blood, and ready to tackle the heavy weights. All my subsequent sets are to failure.

(Continued on page 40)

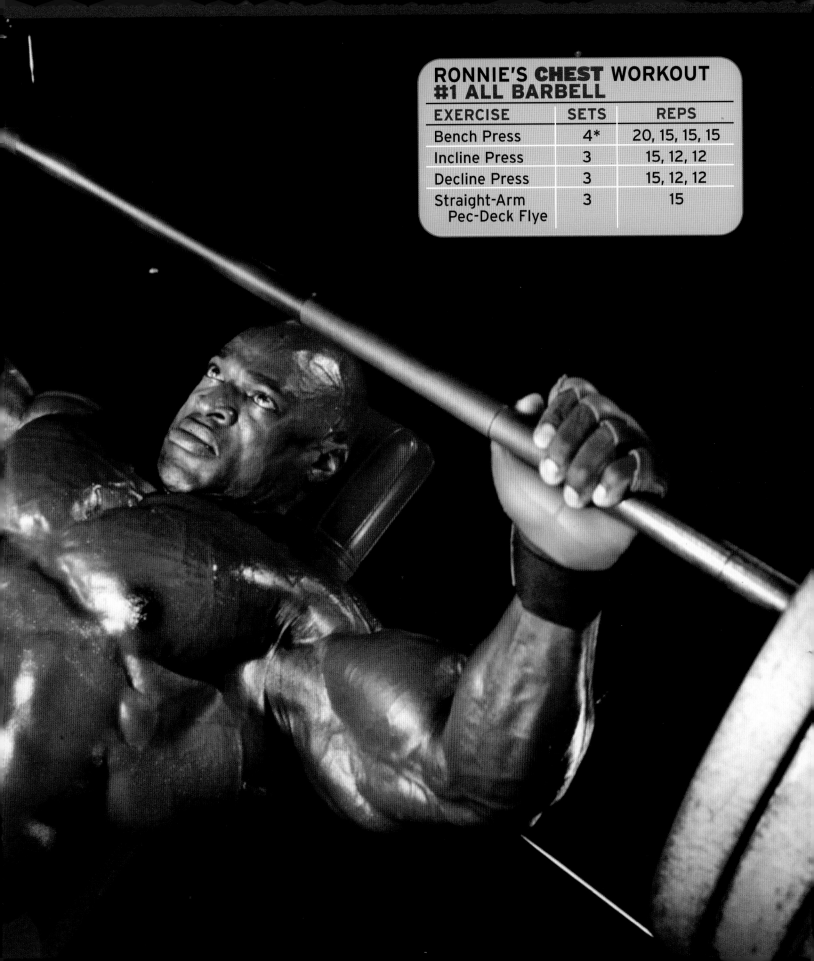

RONNIE'S CHEST WORKOUT
#1 ALL BARBELL

EXERCISE	SETS	REPS
Bench Press	4*	20, 15, 15, 15
Incline Press	3	15, 12, 12
Decline Press	3	15, 12, 12
Straight-Arm Pec-Deck Flye	3	15

BARBELL BENCH PRESS/ BARBELL INCLINE PRESS

Note: The incline bench is shown here.
START | Using a wider-than-shoulder-width grip, unrack the bar and raise it several inches to arms' length.
ACTION | Lower the weight slowly to the upper chest (mid-chest for the flat bench press). As a powerlifter, I was taught to hold the bar on my chest for a count of two and I still do that — don't bounce at the bottom. From there, explode up and repeat.

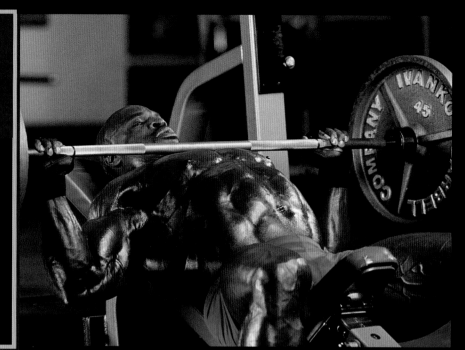

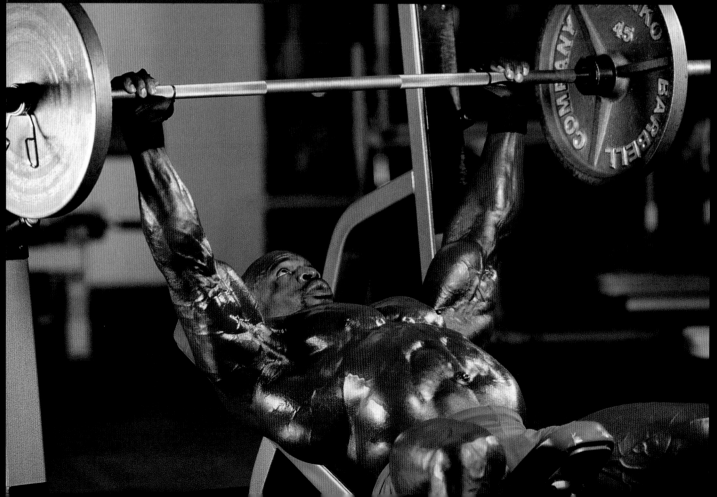

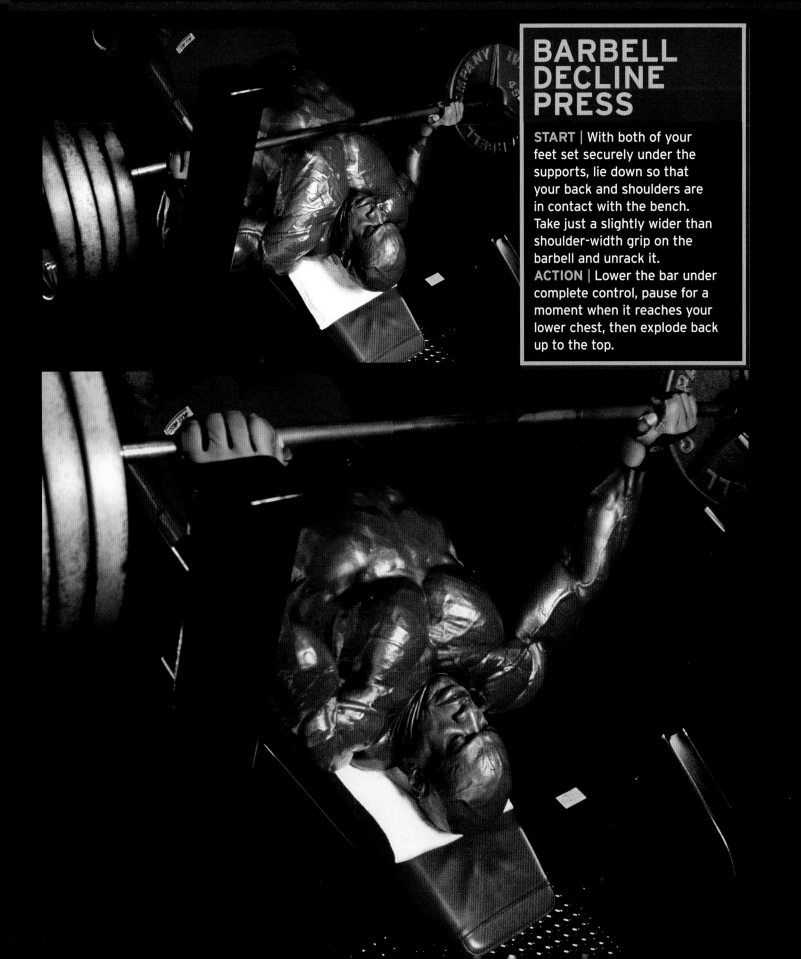

BARBELL DECLINE PRESS

START | With both of your feet set securely under the supports, lie down so that your back and shoulders are in contact with the bench. Take just a slightly wider than shoulder-width grip on the barbell and unrack it.

ACTION | Lower the bar under complete control, pause for a moment when it reaches your lower chest, then explode back up to the top.

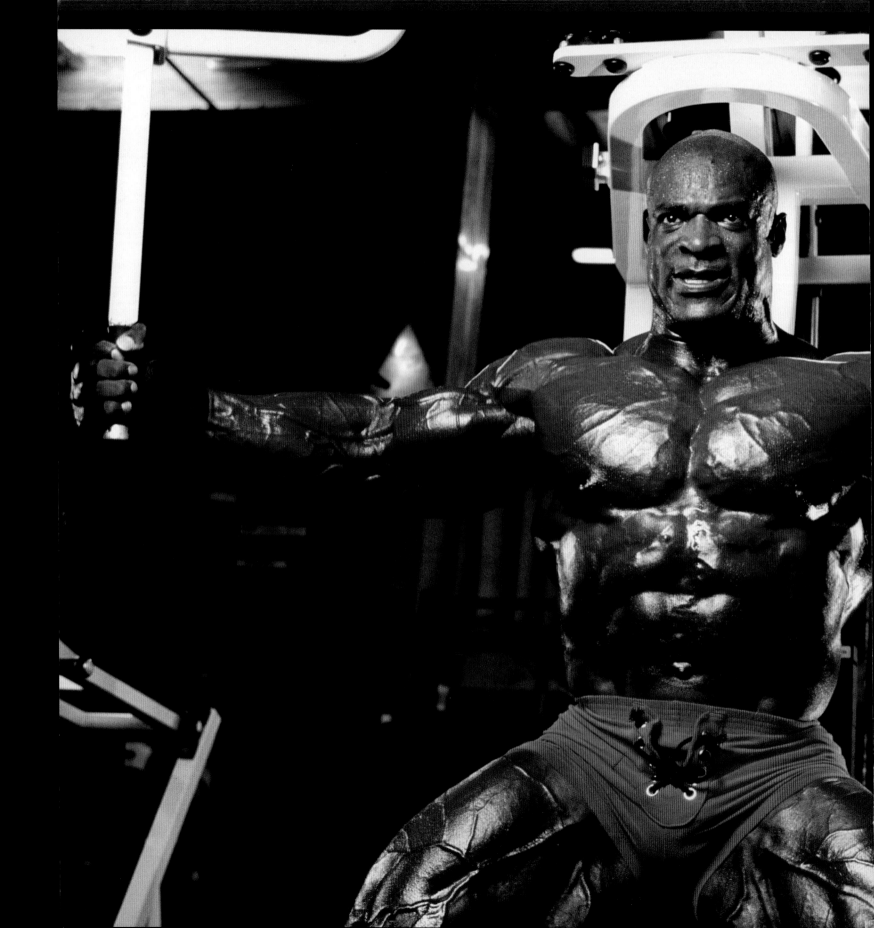

STRAIGHT-ARM PEC DECK FLYE

START | With your back against the pad of the machine, grasp the handles and raise your elbows so they're even with your shoulders and pointed behind you.

ACTION | Keeping your arms straight with just a slight bend in your elbows, flex your pecs hard to bring the handles together in front of your chest. Squeeze – try to press your pecs so hard they rise up and meet in the center of your ribcage – and hold for a strong contraction. Retrace the arc to fully stretch your pecs. This machine also comes with a bent-arm variation, in which you place your elbows and upper arms against a pad. That version works just as well, as long as you concentrate on a powerful contraction within your pectorals as you move through the arc.

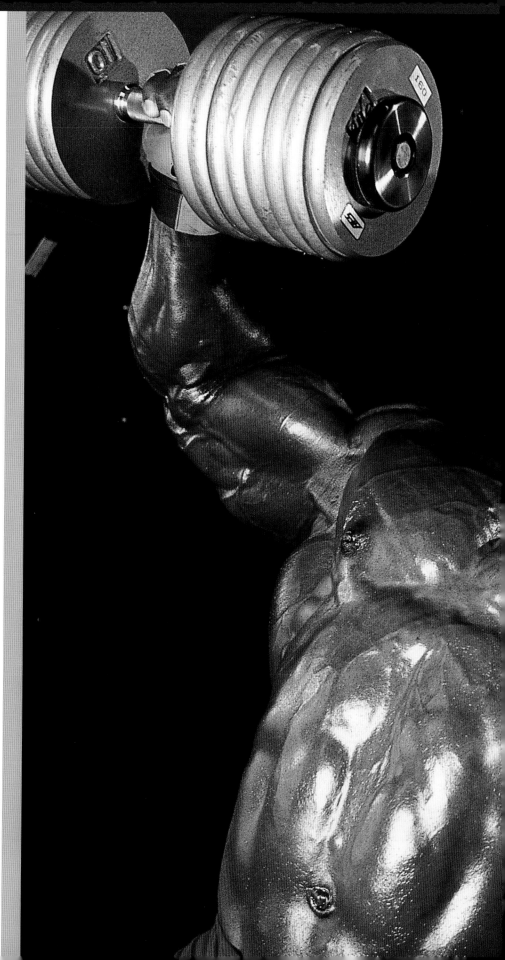

FOR ALL BEGINNER-LEVEL AND INTERMEDIATE BODY-builders, I believe in doing a warm-up set for every chest exercise, not just the first one as I do. This way, you can minimize your risk of injury and really get a feel for the weights before dropping the tonnage on 'em.

I always smash out four chest exercises per workout, whether it's barbell day or dumbbell day. While a beginner should limit themselves to one or two exercises per bodypart, perhaps one press and one flye, I don't see any reason why an intermediate bodybuilder — someone who has trained regularly at least 3–6 months — can't handle four chest exercises per workout. Just taper the weight to your personal strength limits and never skip your warm-up sets.

Another rule of thumb: Do your pressing movements before tackling the flyes. Advanced bodybuilders, who have built all kinds of crazy strength in their pecs over the course of many years, sometimes use a technique called "pre-exhaust" in which you purposely do a flye movement first to tire out the pectorals, then go into your pressing movements while your pecs are somewhat fatigued.

That technique has its place in a weightlifter's tool box, but it's something to be used sparingly, and only if your pecs are so strong that they totally overpower and outlast your triceps. When this happens you may find yourself terminating your pressing sets early because your tri's are fried. For most of you, you'll be best served by sticking to the tried-and-true protocol: Presses (whether incline, flat or decline) come first, flyes (whether dumbbell or machine-based) follow as a finisher.

With that, I give you two of my all-time favorite routines, a chest one-two punch that will knock out boredom and help you pound size mercilessly into your upper, middle and lower pecs.

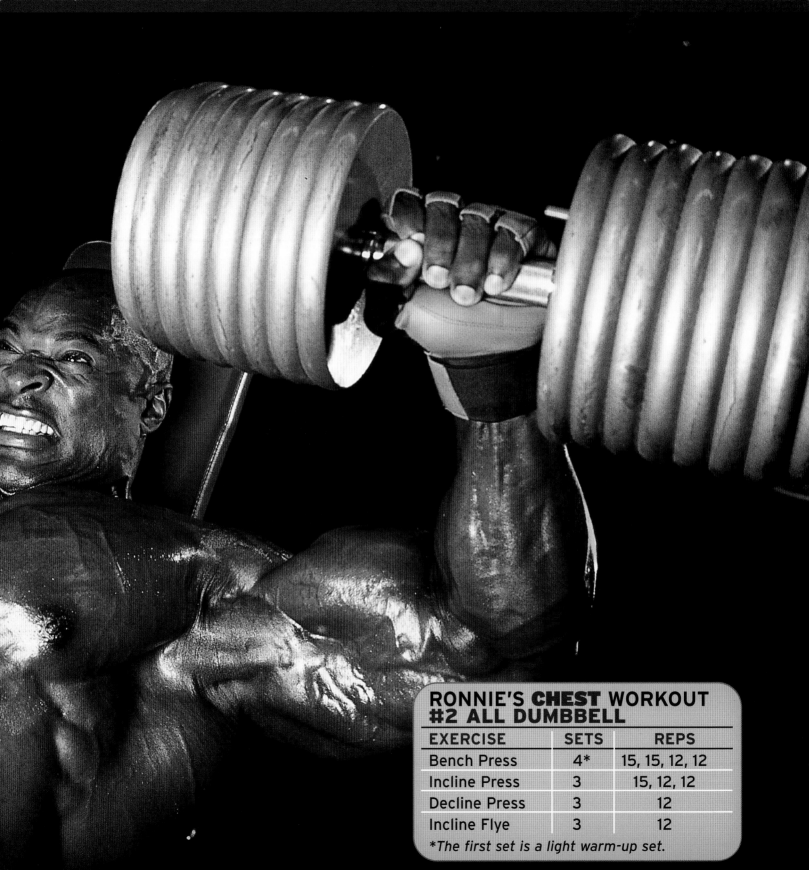

RONNIE'S CHEST WORKOUT
#2 ALL DUMBBELL

EXERCISE	SETS	REPS
Bench Press	4*	15, 15, 12, 12
Incline Press	3	15, 12, 12
Decline Press	3	12
Incline Flye	3	12

*The first set is a light warm-up set.

DUMBBELL BENCH PRESS

START | Lie back on a flat bench with two dumbbells in hand. Hold them at the sides of your chest, elbows out and pointing down.

ACTION | Press the weights up to full extension, touching the dumbbells together at the top. I sometimes use the touching-the-weights-together technique to fully contract my pecs, but this strategy can backfire if you don't use proper form. Control the "tap"; letting the dumbbells clang together as they come toward each other overhead takes stress off of the chest and makes this move much less effective.

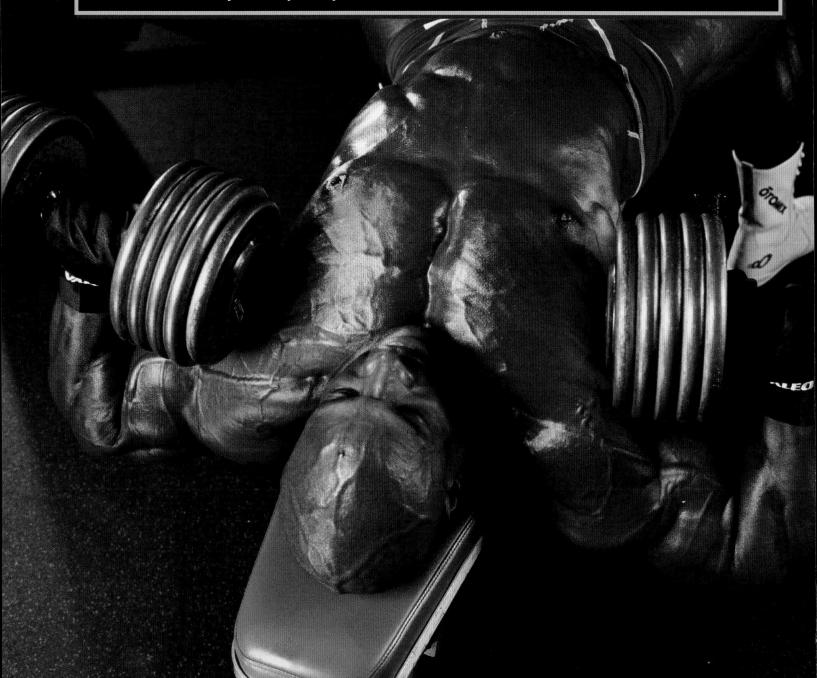

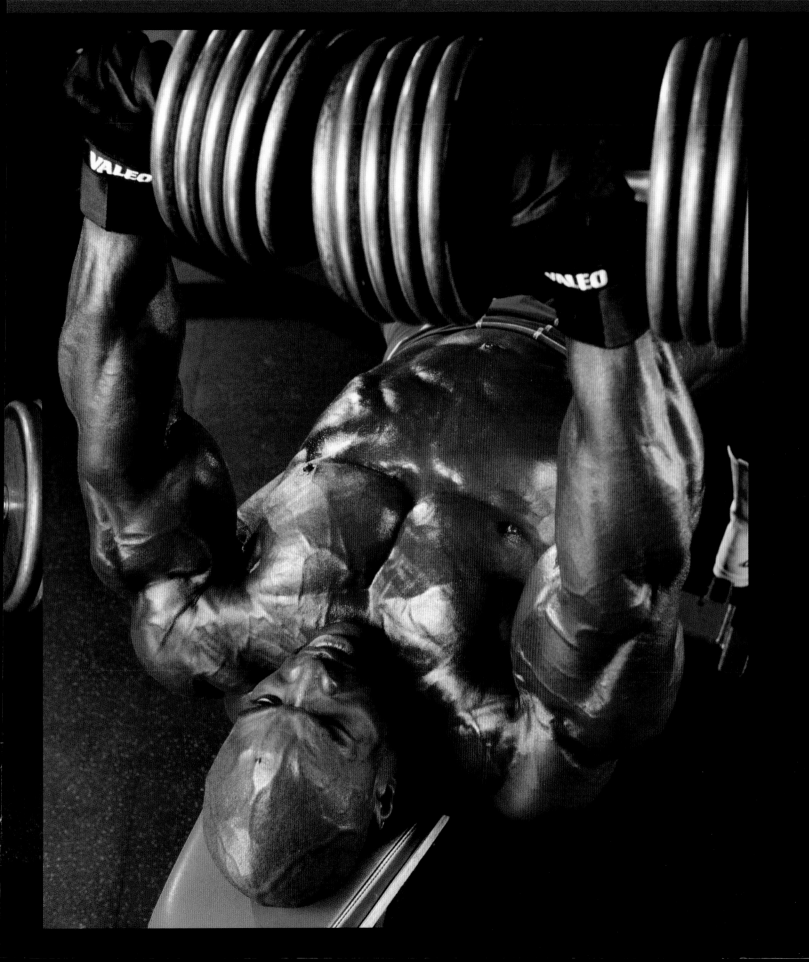

DUMBBELL INCLINE PRESS

START | The start is similar to the flat-bench dumbbell press, except the weights should be more in line with your upper chest in the bottom position.

ACTION | Press the dumbbells forcefully upward, contracting your pecs on the way up. Don't arch your back and squirm on the bench in an effort to lift a weight that's too heavy for you.

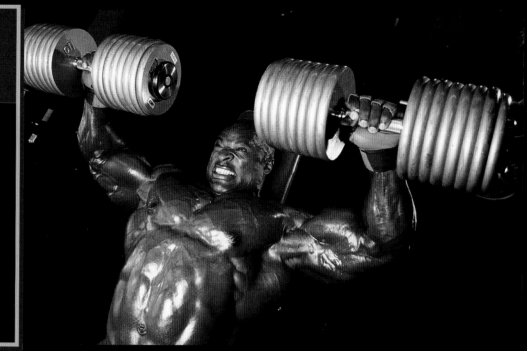

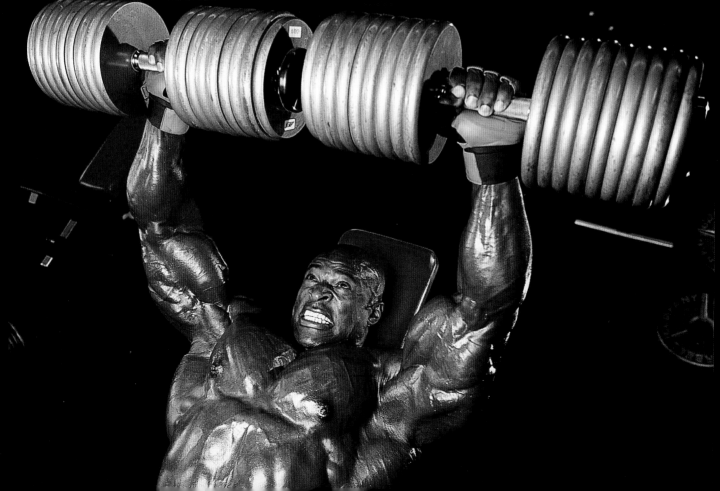

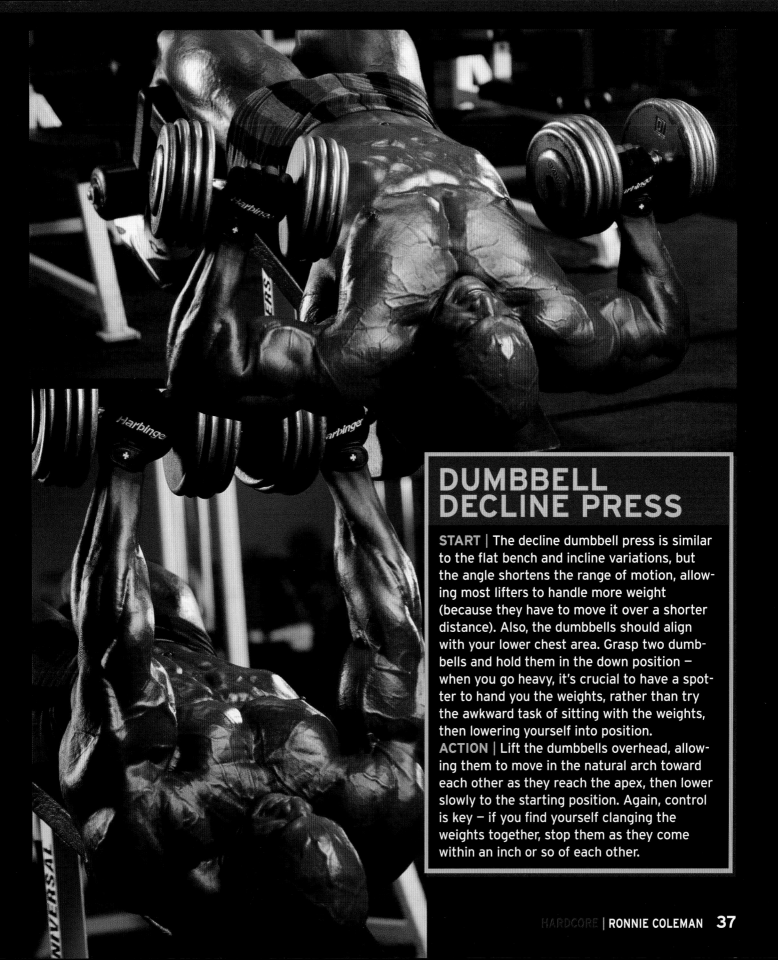

DUMBBELL DECLINE PRESS

START | The decline dumbbell press is similar to the flat bench and incline variations, but the angle shortens the range of motion, allowing most lifters to handle more weight (because they have to move it over a shorter distance). Also, the dumbbells should align with your lower chest area. Grasp two dumbbells and hold them in the down position – when you go heavy, it's crucial to have a spotter to hand you the weights, rather than try the awkward task of sitting with the weights, then lowering yourself into position.

ACTION | Lift the dumbbells overhead, allowing them to move in the natural arch toward each other as they reach the apex, then lower slowly to the starting position. Again, control is key – if you find yourself clanging the weights together, stop them as they come within an inch or so of each other.

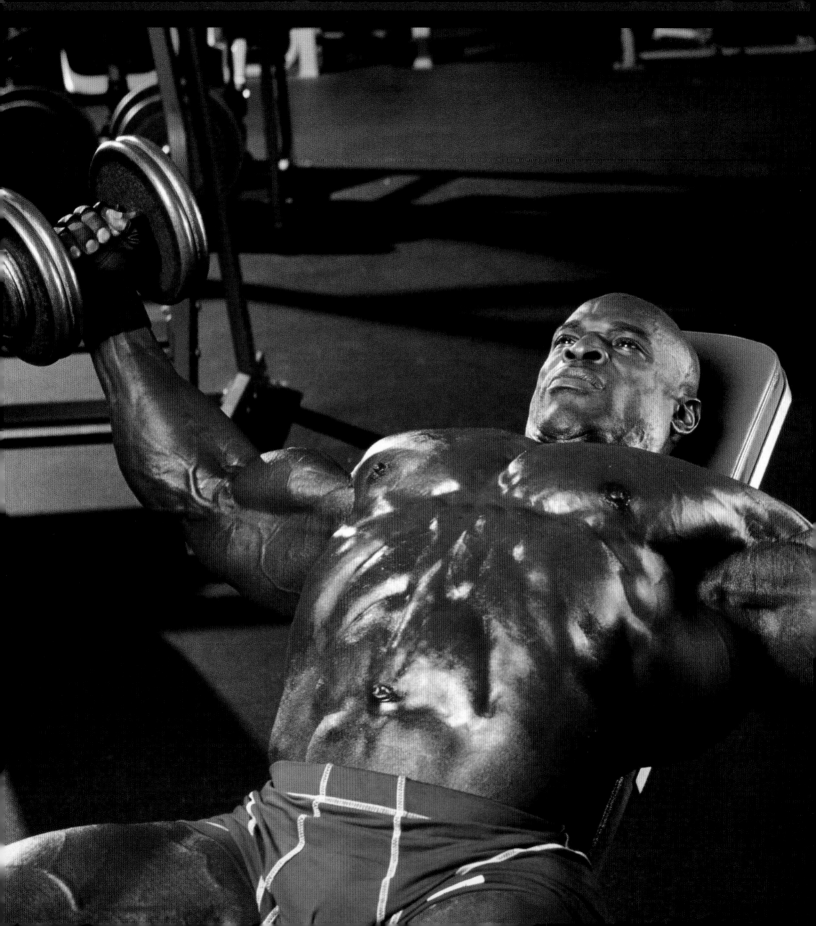

INCLINE DUMBBELL FLYE

START | Hold the dumbbells straight overhead, elbows barely bent to protect the joint from over-extension.

ACTION | Lower the weights in an arc out to each side until they reach chest level. Using the old "hugging a tree" adage, retrace the movement to return to the dumbbells-overhead position. I see a lot of guys who don't lower the weights out and down far enough to get a full stretch, which is a must. As with dumbbell presses, you can touch the weights at the top and squeeze them together for that killer contraction, but control is essential – bang them together, and you risk injuring yourself while introducing unwanted momentum to the lift.

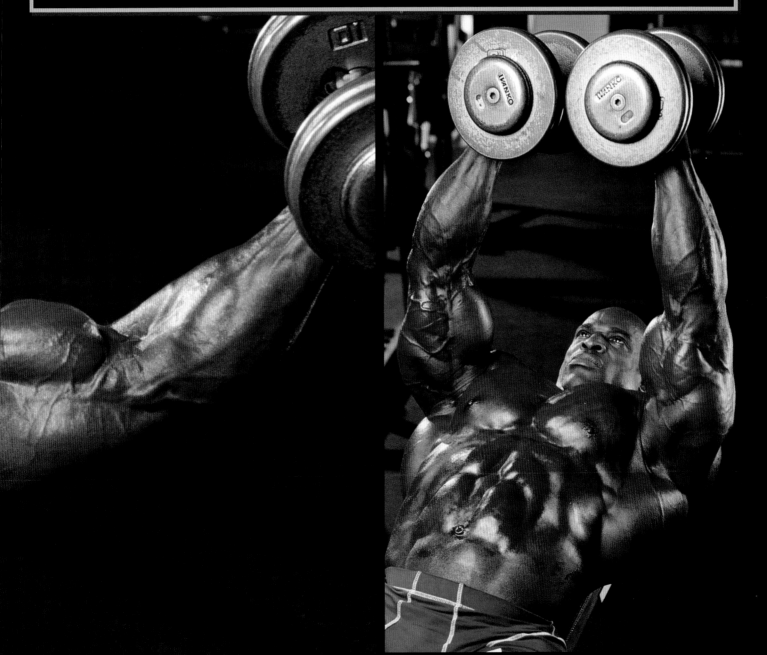

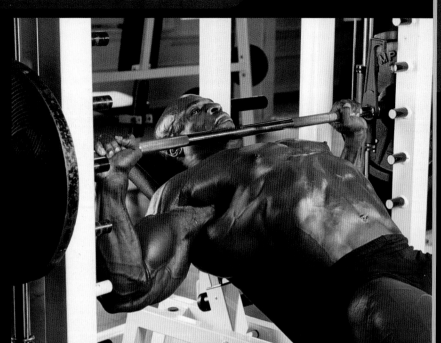

SMITH-MACHINE INCLINE PRESS

START | The Smith machine is a solid instrument to use if you want to go all-out on a press – you don't have to worry as much about balancing the bar, since the apparatus does it for you. To begin, center an incline bench in the machine at a point where the bar comes down to your upper pecs (you should "test" it, pressing with the bar only to make sure it's placed correctly).

ACTION | Grasp the bar with an overhand grip, unhook it from the supports, bring it down to your chest, then push forcefully to full extension. Lower and repeat.

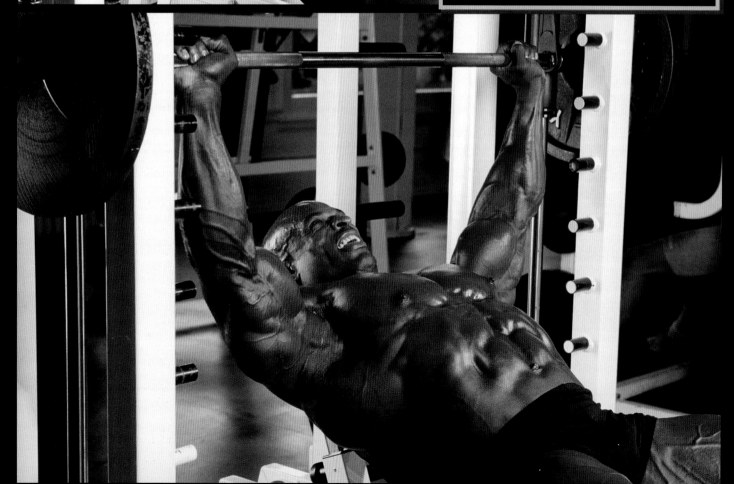

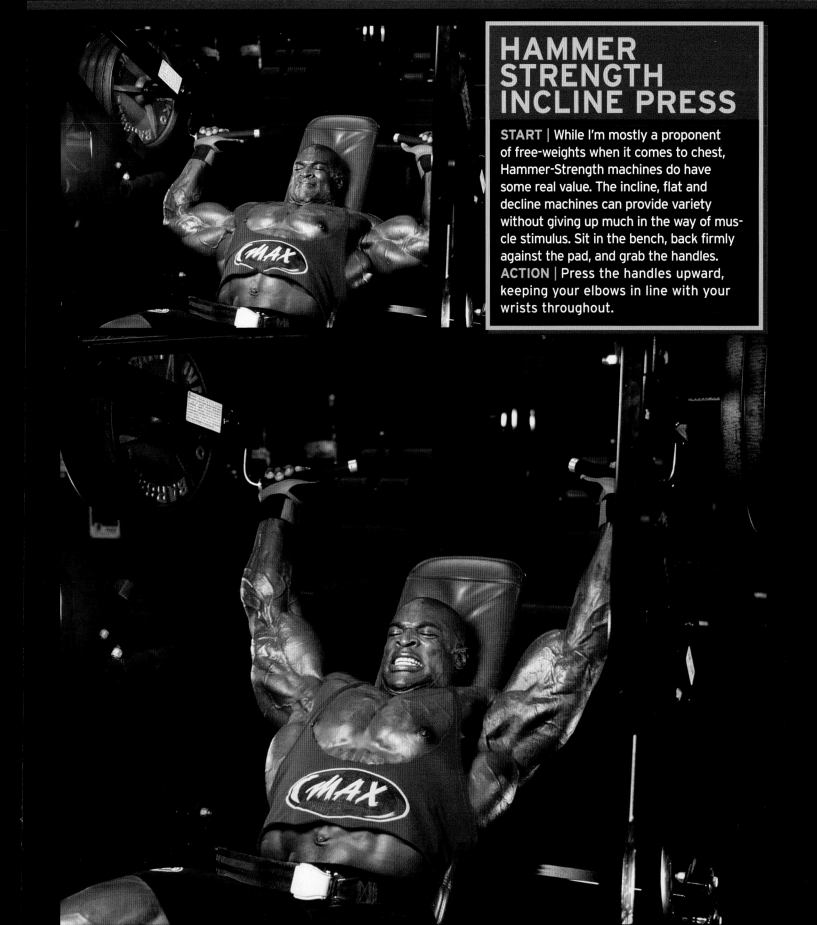

HAMMER STRENGTH INCLINE PRESS

START | While I'm mostly a proponent of free-weights when it comes to chest, Hammer-Strength machines do have some real value. The incline, flat and decline machines can provide variety without giving up much in the way of muscle stimulus. Sit in the bench, back firmly against the pad, and grab the handles. **ACTION** | Press the handles upward, keeping your elbows in line with your wrists throughout.

Ronnie's Chest Lessons

1 HAVE YOU HIT A STICKING POINT in your presses? Try benching in a power rack. Here's how it works: Set the flat, incline or decline bench (whichever you need help with) in the power rack, then set the stopper bars a few inches above your chest (where your chest would be while you're laying on the bench). Place a barbell in the rack, load it up and do some heavy sets. For instance, do three sets of five reps each of the heaviest weight you can handle (perhaps a weight you've been struggling with). At the bottom of each rep, instead of coming down to your chest, you'll be coming down and resting on the support bars, then pressing with all your might from that point. This way, you don't get stuck at the bottom, you get used to handling that heavy weight, and you build strength so that once you go back to the regular barbell press after a few weeks of the power-rack variation, you should be able to get beyond that sticking point.

2 ROTATE WHICH PRESS you start with on a workout-to-workout basis. Don't get in the habit of always starting with incline, or flat, or whatever version of the bench happens to be your favorite. Your first exercise is the one you can give the most energy to, so you want to hit a different area of your chest while you're freshest each time. One week, start with flat-bench presses. Next time, do the inclines first. This advice is especially valid for beginners, but even advanced athletes need this kind of variation for best results.

3 ON YOUR FLYE MOVES, there are two different hand positions you can try. The traditional way to do a dumbbell flye is with your palms facing each other. However, you can also do flyes with your palms down (thumbs facing each other). Some people find this position more comfortable, and can even move a little bit more weight than with the palms-facing version. In this game, the more weight you can work with under control, the more strength and size you can build. Experiment and find which way is more comfortable for you, and go with it.

4 ONE WAY TO SHOCK yourself out of a training rut when it comes to your pecs is to throw a workout at your body that it's not accustomed to. It's not necessary to go to the extremes of some grueling marathon session where you pound your chest with every conceivable exercise — in fact, that could be counterproductive, as it's essentially overtraining. Instead, a shock can come from something as simple as changing up your workouts so one day is all presses, the next session is all flyes. Try that for a few weeks and go back to your regular sessions. Or combine your workout into compound sets, such as this: a barbell bench press/flat-bench flye to start, 3-4 sets of 10-15 reps each exercise, followed by a decline Smith-machine press/decline dumbbell flye compound set for the same set and rep scheme. You don't need to reinvent the wheel for shock, just tweak it a bit to get gains rolling.

5 ANOTHER "SHOCKING" TRICK: the rest-pause technique. In rest-pause, you take breaks within a set in order to extend a set beyond your normal capacity. This is how it works: Say you're on the Hammer-Strength press machine. Start with your set, going to 10 reps or more, as many as you can get without stopping. When you reach a point of momentary muscular failure, pause — either in the top position or bottom — and rest for about five seconds. Then continue the set, trying to get at least 2-3 more reps. At that point, you can either terminate the set, or rest and try again to pump out a few more. The technique takes advantage of a muscle's fast recovery time — upon failing, muscles recover at least a portion of their strength within seconds. Rest-pause isn't limited to your chest workouts; feel free to use this in any of your bodypart training. Just don't go overboard and use it every single workout, or even every week. Too much, and you'll quickly enter a state of overtraining.

6 MANY LIFTERS SHARE a common problem: Their upper chest is shallow and lags well behind their bigger middle pecs. If this describes your current condition, consider making one of your two chest workouts each week an "all-upper" day. Start with incline barbell or dumbbell presses, do a Hammer Strength or other type of machine incline press second, and finish with dumbbell or cable incline flyes. For each exercise, do four sets, 10-15 reps per set.

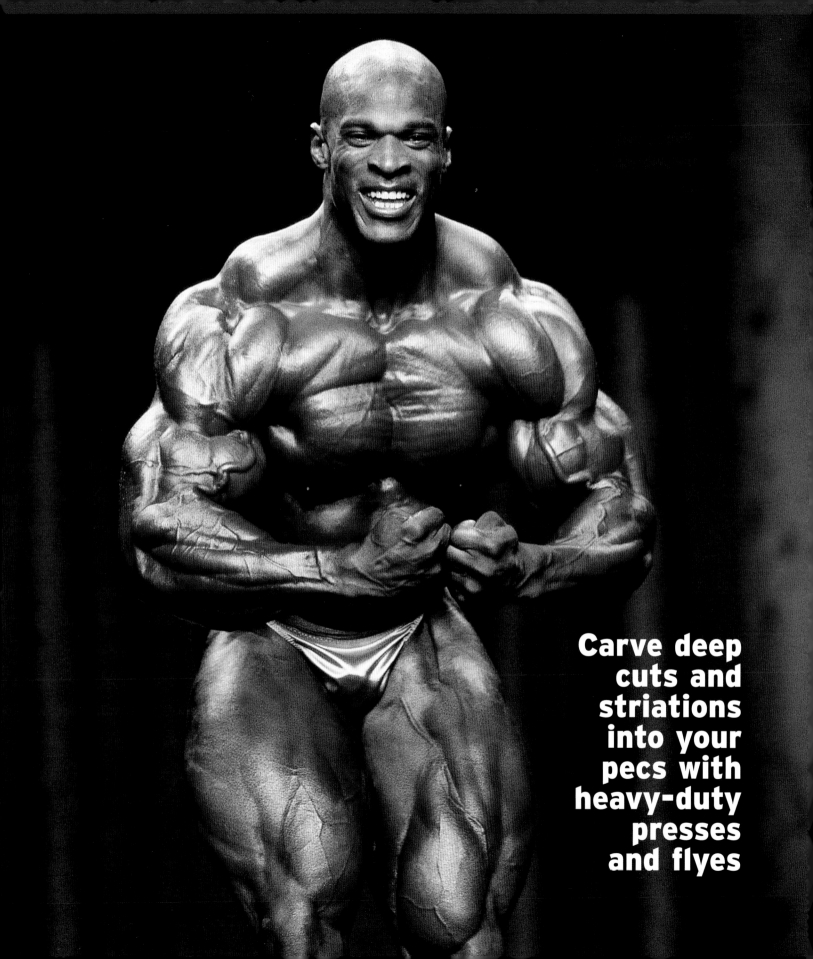

Carve deep cuts and striations into your pecs with heavy-duty presses and flyes

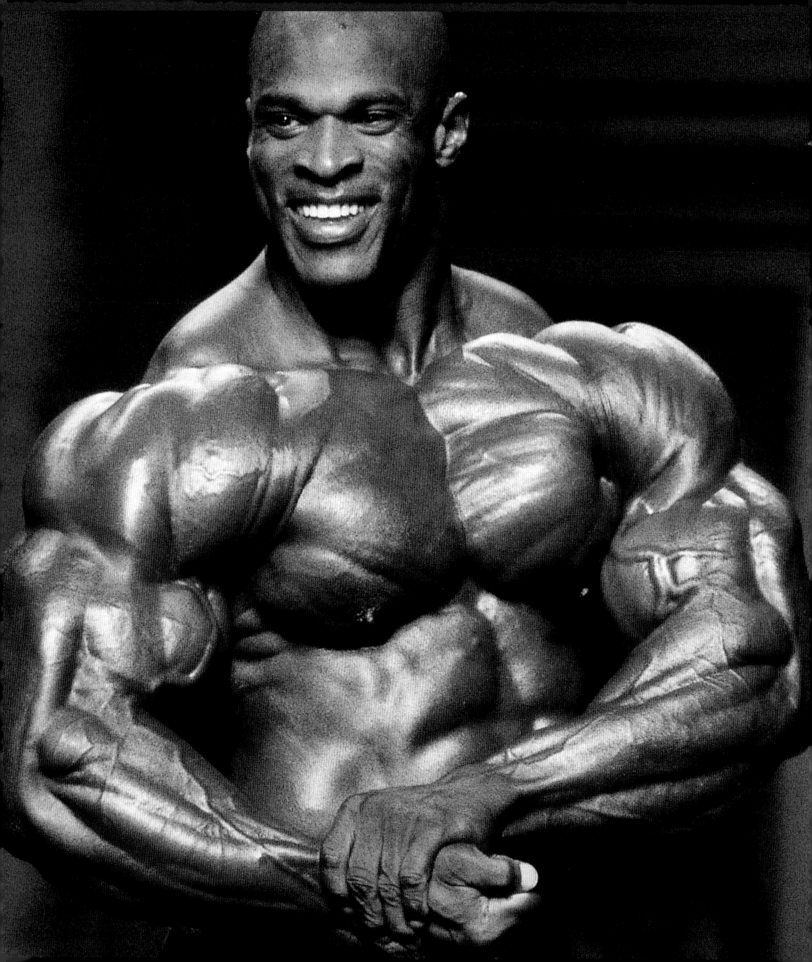

7 WOULD YOU LIKE A very simple way to increase your power on your bench press? Take a stronger grip on the bar! Just by putting a little extra oomph in your grip, you'll find you can handle a bit more poundage. This might work because you're consciously tensing your body a bit more by doing so, but whatever the physiological mechanism may be, just try it and you'll see – it works.

8 DUMBBELL PRESSES may be the "perfect" chest exercise, if there is such a thing. Even if you're not going to do my twice-per-week, barbell and dumbbell workout days as I prescribe, you should at the very least make sure you do some form of dumbbell press regularly in your chest training. My three most hallowed training principles are: 1) use the most weight possible, 2) with the correct form, 3) through a full range of motion. Nothing in chest training comes closer to satisfying all three criteria than dumbbell presses. On a machine or with a barbell, you're limited in the stretch at the bottom, and your range of motion at the top; neither of which is an issue with dumbbells. Also, by pressing the dumbbells together at the top in a controlled manner, I can squeeze hard enough that my pecs pop upward like mountain peaks, driving hardness and definition through every inch of those muscles.

9 IF YOU HAVE THE ADVANTAGE OF A BENCH that adjusts to multiple angles in a range between upright and decline, don't be afraid to use all the angles available. In other words, you don't have to use the same exact incline or decline setting every week on your dumbbell presses, nor should you: Even little variations in your incline or decline can make a decided difference in what fibers you're hitting week to week. You want to hit as many new fibers as possible over the course of a month, a year and beyond. Of course, if all you have is benches that don't adjust, that's fine, but if you have adjustable equipment, use it to its full capacity.

10 TO BURN OUT ANY last remaining muscle left untouched by your workout, you can add a bodyweight exercise such as push-ups to failure as your final set. No fancy technique here, just drop to the floor and give yourself 20, or as many as your fatigue will allow before you collapse in a heap. You can also do parallel-bar dips, but be sure to perform the version where you angle your torso forward, which tags the chest muscles more than the straight-up type of dip. (Crossing your ankles and bending your knees will help shift your weight enough to achieve the desired angle in your body.)

11 ISOMETRIC FLEXING between sets is a way to create more muscle density and hardness over the long haul. If you aspire to become a competitive bodybuilder, flexing your working muscles for a 10-count (or more) between sets is also a good way to learn control and to practice holding a pose. Anyone who thinks posing is easy ought to try it – I'd argue you could get a great workout just by practicing posing. Go through a bonafide bodybuilding show and you'll know, nothing is as draining as holding poses as hard as you can under the scrutiny of judges for hours on end. Take this advice too far and you're bound to lose steam as your workout goes on, but if you try it on a limited basis, throwing in perhaps one or two 10-second poses during the course of each exercise, you shouldn't compromise your strength too greatly.

12 ON PRESSING MOVES, do you find that you reflexively bring in your elbows tight to the sides of your body? That's a sign that your triceps are overpowering your pectoral muscles. You want to keep your elbows away from your body, so your arm forms a 90-degree angle to your torso in order to keep the stress squarely on the pecs where it belongs. Also, stack your wrists over your elbows – in other words, make sure your elbows stay directly under your wrist joint, which gives you more driving power as you press.

13 AS YOU CAN SEE from the selection of chest moves in this chapter, there are only two effective ways to work your pectorals – with a flye and with a press. It's not rocket science, so don't try to make your quest for a better chest more complicated than it needs to be. Stick to basic bread-and-butter exercises; don't try to get too clever. I always see guys in the gym trying some crazy stuff, but bottom line, if you ain't pressin' or flyin', your chest ain't workin.'

CHAPTER 4
EXPAND YOUR
THIGHS

Do you have stick legs or tree trunks? The answer to that question separates the men from the boys in the gym. If you're only half serious about training, chances are you don't give much thought or time to your legs. Perhaps you only perform a half-hearted set of leg extensions and curls here and there to break up your chest and arm days.

If that describes you, it's not too late. Hey, you picked up this book, after all. If you're ready to get serious, this is the workout that'll get you on track. Don't be the guy with the scrawny legs at the gym anymore – be the guy that sets the standard for intensity and excellence. And you don't need a Mr. Olympia title to do that.

LEAD OFF MY WORKOUT with leg extensions, not only to warm up my quads but also to pre-exhaust them before the heavier, compound exercises like squats, leg presses and lunges. I can't over-emphasize the importance of warming up your knees, quads and heart rate, especially considering what's to follow. Start with four sets of leg extensions, 15–30 reps each. Every set should be with the same weight, but put enough plates on the stack so that by the fourth set, it becomes a working exercise in which you're struggling to get your 30 reps. Range of motion is full and continuously tensed; get a hard, peak-contraction squeeze at the top of each repetition.

Next up, squats. Since I don't like the controlled pulley action of a Smith machine, and dumbbells are just too light to really give me a challenge, I stick to barbells for all my squats. Although I'm pretty warm by now, I still do another warm-up set of 20 reps of the squat to ensure that my quads are ready for a pounding, then four pyramided sets, 10–15 reps each, the last one to failure. As for your stance on this exercise, don't go so wide that your hips are stressed and not so close that you lose stability.

On my third exercise, I choose between hack squats or leg presses. No further warm-up is needed, so start with enough weight to get a good burn with 15 reps on your first set, then keep pyramiding up on your second set and your third, this latter one all-out to failure. Now, add even more weight and do another set for 10–12, again to absolute failure. Don't cheat with partial reps; use a full range of motion and constant tension.

Lying leg curls to focus directly on my hamstrings come fourth, and I finish with walking lunges. I often hit the gym parking lot and lunge across it. Try this, and whether you're in the Texas heat like me or not, and you'll fry your thigh muscles — but that sweet burn you're guaranteed to feel leads to some amazing results.

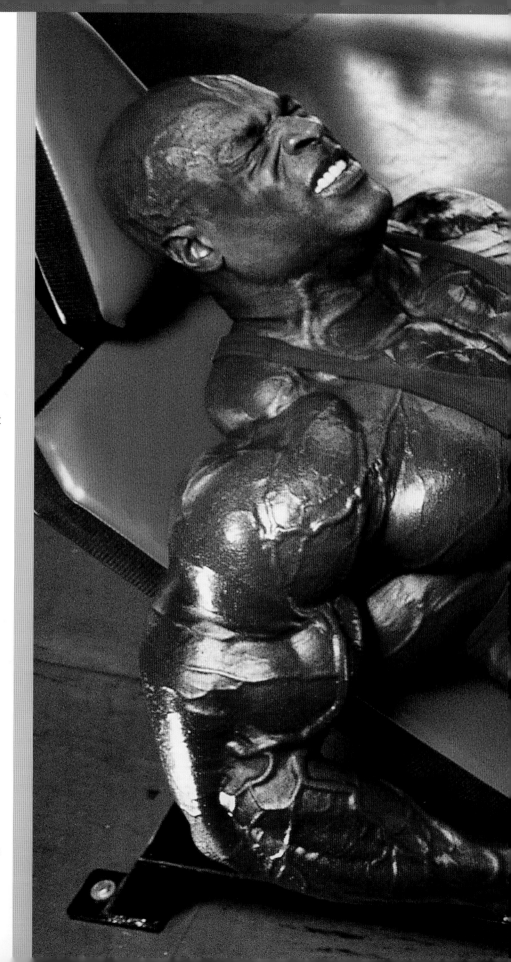

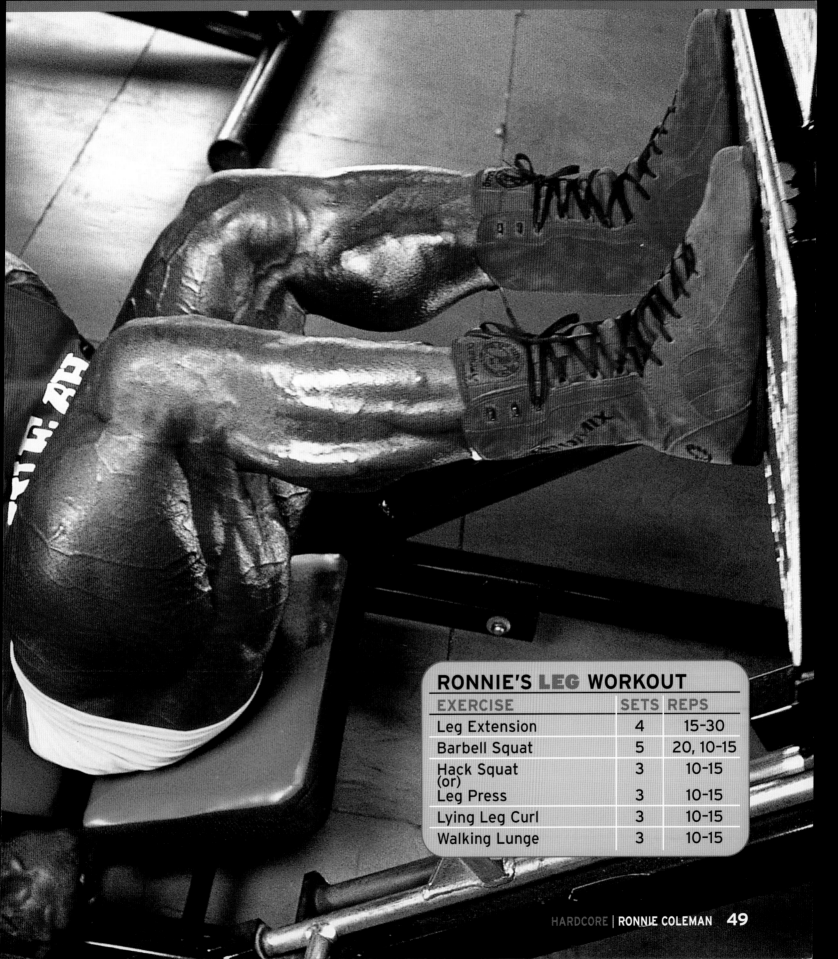

RONNIE'S LEG WORKOUT

EXERCISE	SETS	REPS
Leg Extension	4	15-30
Barbell Squat	5	20, 10-15
Hack Squat (or)	3	10-15
Leg Press	3	10-15
Lying Leg Curl	3	10-15
Walking Lunge	3	10-15

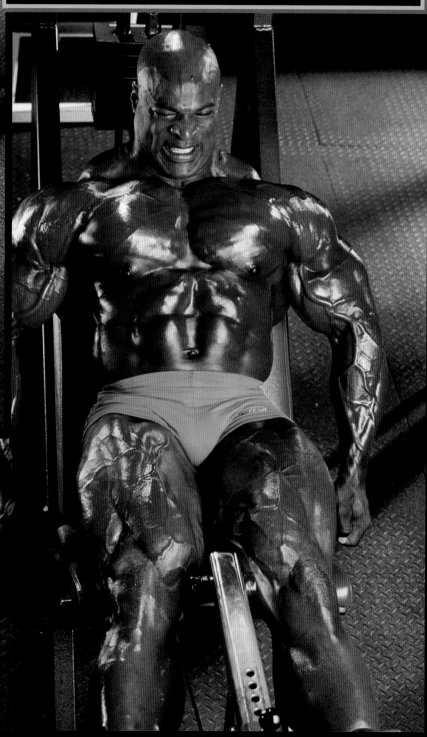

LEG EXTENSION

START | Adjust a leg extension machine so your thighs are fully supported right up to your knees. The foot roller should rest on or just above your ankles.

ACTION | Grasp the handles on either side of the seat and slowly contract through your quads to raise the weight stack. Pause a moment at the top before slowly lowering the stack back to the start, and go right into the next repetition.

If you can max out the weight stack of the machine, try doing extensions one leg at a time instead

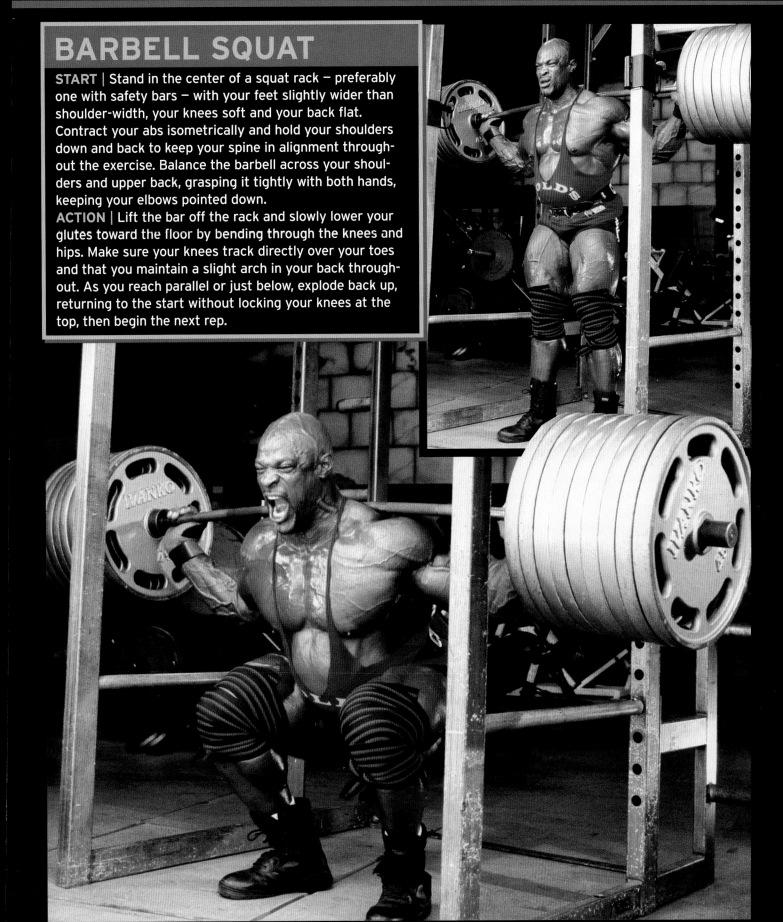

BARBELL SQUAT

START | Stand in the center of a squat rack – preferably one with safety bars – with your feet slightly wider than shoulder-width, your knees soft and your back flat. Contract your abs isometrically and hold your shoulders down and back to keep your spine in alignment throughout the exercise. Balance the barbell across your shoulders and upper back, grasping it tightly with both hands, keeping your elbows pointed down.

ACTION | Lift the bar off the rack and slowly lower your glutes toward the floor by bending through the knees and hips. Make sure your knees track directly over your toes and that you maintain a slight arch in your back throughout. As you reach parallel or just below, explode back up, returning to the start without locking your knees at the top, then begin the next rep.

HACK SQUAT

START | A lot of people shy away from the hack squat machine in favor of the leg press exclusively, and that's a shame. It's true, the hack squat is harder – if you doubt me, think for a second how much weight you can push on the press vs. the hack squat – but that challenge is what makes it beneficial. Adjust a hack squat machine so that the pads rest comfortably on your shoulders, and your back and neck are fully supported. I place my toes toward the top of the platform to make sure I hit my upper quads as much as possible. I also stand with my feet shoulder-width apart. Some people stand with them closer together, but the closer they are, the more you start to use your inner thighs.

ACTION | Unhook the safety handles and slowly squat down toward the platform, keeping your knees directly over your toes on the descent. If you let your knees shift to one side or the other, you put unnecessary shearing stress on the ligaments and tendons of your knees. As you reach parallel or just below, reverse the motion and press back up to the start. Without locking out your knees, begin the next repetition. On this exercise, like squats, it's helpful to think about "driving through your heels" to press yourself back up to a standing position; this mental trick helps engage the glutes, quadriceps and hamstrings to generate the power you need to finish each repetition.

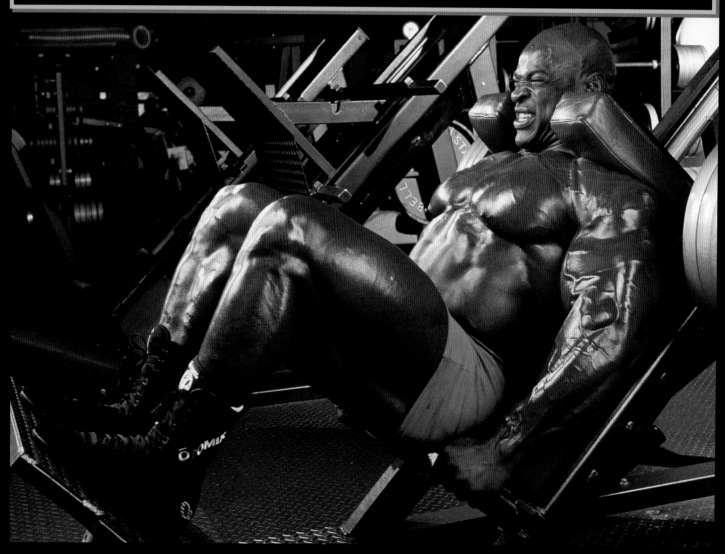

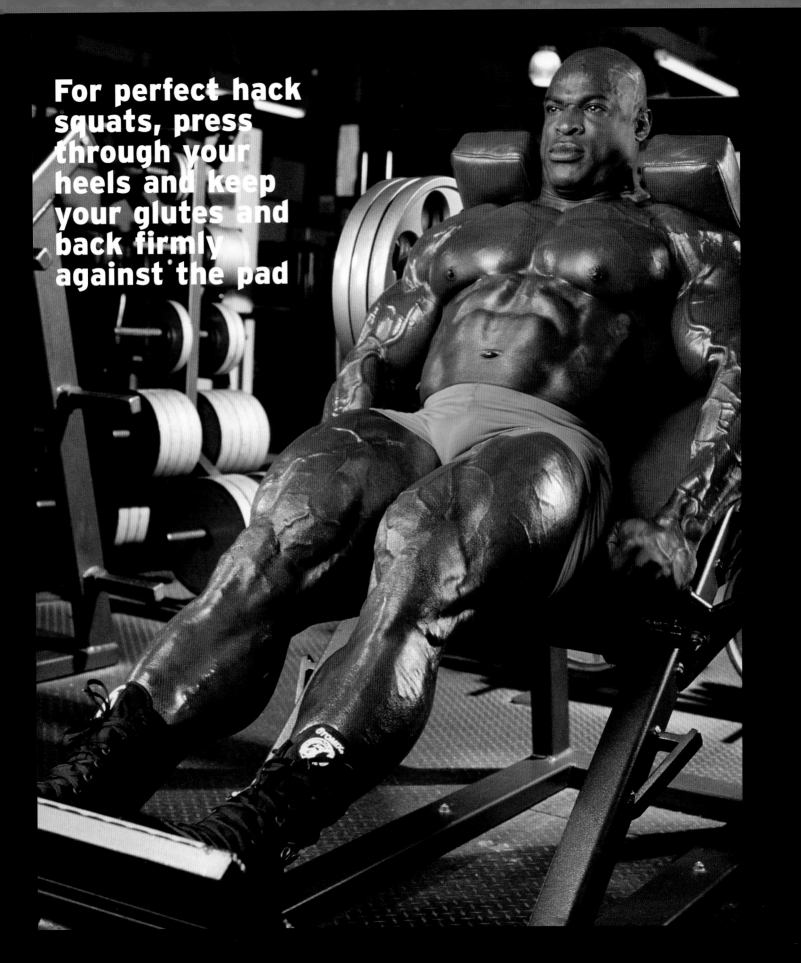

For perfect hack squats, press through your heels and keep your glutes and back firmly against the pad

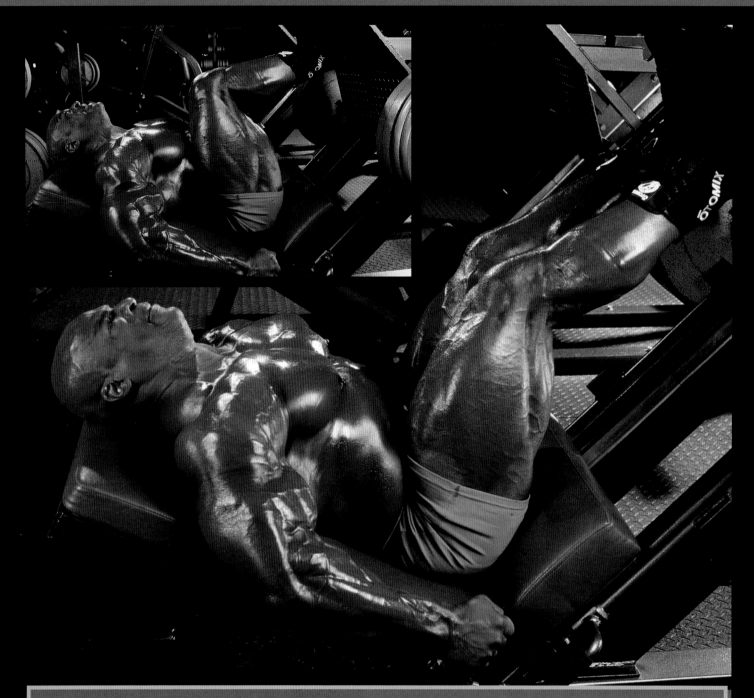

LEG PRESS

START | Sit in a leg press machine and press your lower back into the seat cushion. My feet are a little less than shoulder-width apart for these so I really feel it in the upper and outer parts of my quads. Unhook the safety latches, then grasp the handles on the machine for stability.

ACTION | Slowly lower the cart toward you while keeping your feet flat on the cart surface. As your knees approach your chest, reverse the motion and press the weight explosively back up to the top. Go right into the next repetition. Don't put your hands on your knees to help move the weight up.

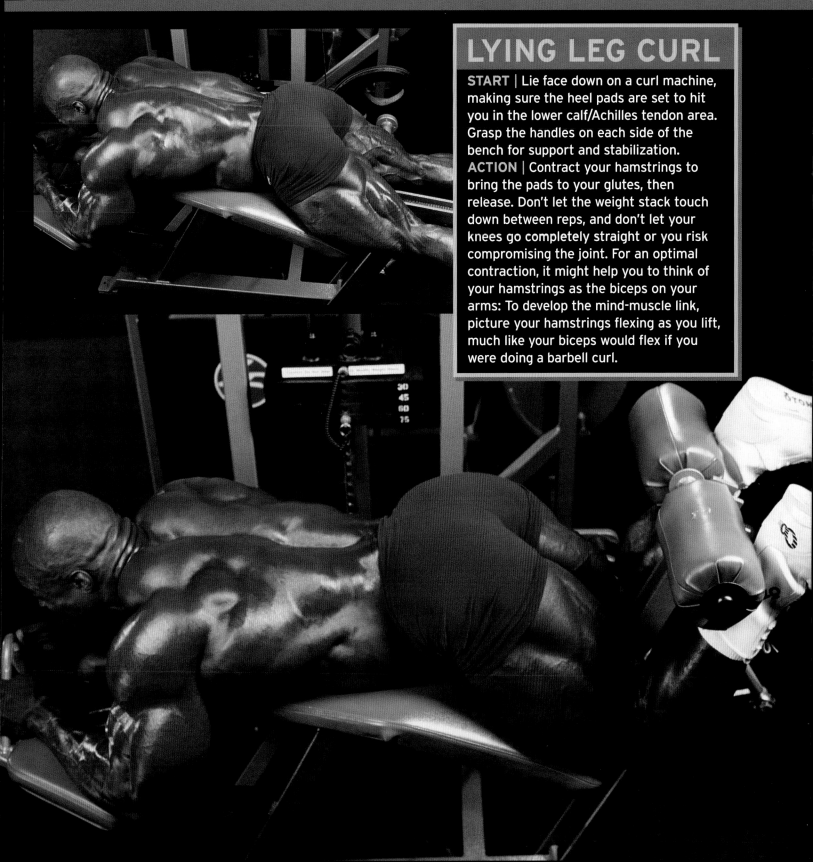

LYING LEG CURL

START | Lie face down on a curl machine, making sure the heel pads are set to hit you in the lower calf/Achilles tendon area. Grasp the handles on each side of the bench for support and stabilization.

ACTION | Contract your hamstrings to bring the pads to your glutes, then release. Don't let the weight stack touch down between reps, and don't let your knees go completely straight or you risk compromising the joint. For an optimal contraction, it might help you to think of your hamstrings as the biceps on your arms: To develop the mind-muscle link, picture your hamstrings flexing as you lift, much like your biceps would flex if you were doing a barbell curl.

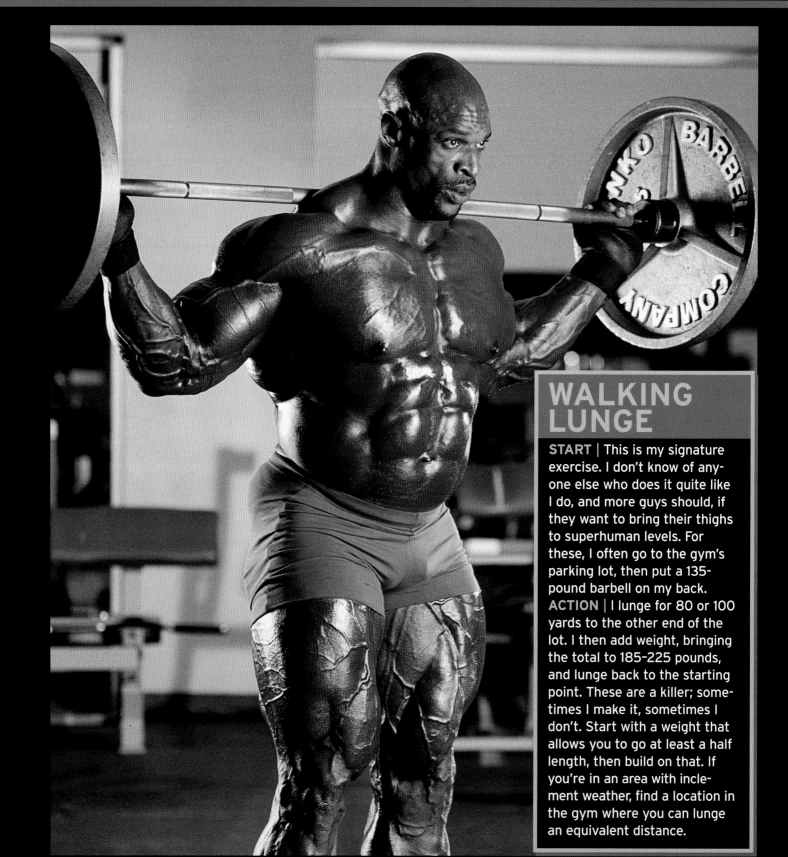

WALKING LUNGE

START | This is my signature exercise. I don't know of anyone else who does it quite like I do, and more guys should, if they want to bring their thighs to superhuman levels. For these, I often go to the gym's parking lot, then put a 135-pound barbell on my back.

ACTION | I lunge for 80 or 100 yards to the other end of the lot. I then add weight, bringing the total to 185–225 pounds, and lunge back to the starting point. These are a killer; sometimes I make it, sometimes I don't. Start with a weight that allows you to go at least a half length, then build on that. If you're in an area with inclement weather, find a location in the gym where you can lunge an equivalent distance.

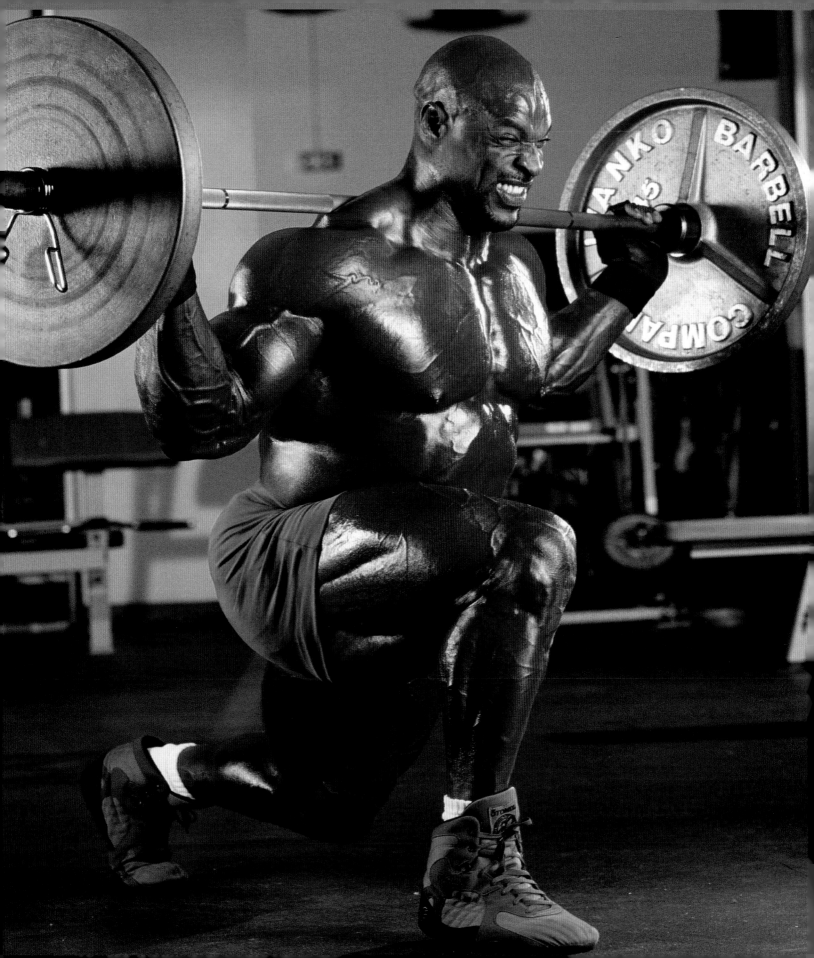

Final Notes

On the next three pages, you'll find three solid hamstring exercises, which you can use in place of lying leg curls whenever you're looking to change up your workout a bit.

You may notice I don't have specific calf exercises listed in this leg workout. I hit calves at least twice per week, tacking them on to the end of a workout — sometimes on leg day, sometimes another day.

When it comes to calves, there isn't any "magical" exercise — standing calf raises, leg-press calf raises, seated calf raises (shown on page 71) and donkey calf raises are the four moves in which you get the most bang for your buck. Choose two of those, making sure to work in seated raises at least every other calf workout (they target the soleus muscle on the back of your lower leg, a muscle that the other three moves don't work); perform four sets, 15–30 reps, going as heavy as you possibly can while moving through a full range of motion.

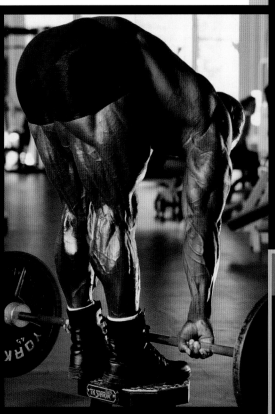

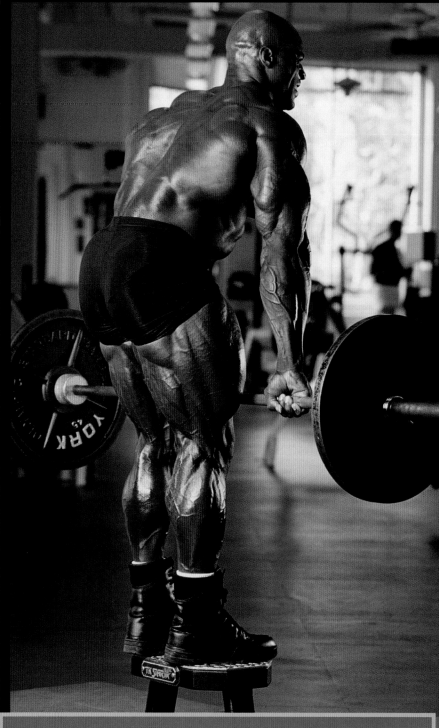

ROMANIAN DEADLIFT

START | For this hamstrings exercise, stand on a platform or the floor, holding a barbell with a shoulder-width, overhand grip.
ACTION | Simultaneously bend over, press your hips back and slide the bar down the front of your thighs to a point between your kneecap and your feet, depending on your flexibility. As you come up, think about driving your feet into the platform or floor, pressing your hips forward and squeezing your glutes.

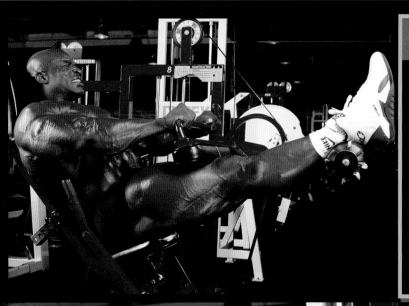

SEATED LEG CURL

START | Adjust the ankle pad of a seated curl machine so it hits just above your Achilles tendons. Sit down, making sure your glutes and lower back are in solid contact with the seat.

ACTION | Curl both legs to a point beneath you, stopping where the machine's range of motion ends or at a point just past a 90-degree angle at your knees. Squeeze your hams for 1–2 seconds, then slowly allow your lower legs to return to the start. Stop before the weight stack touches down and begin the next repetition.

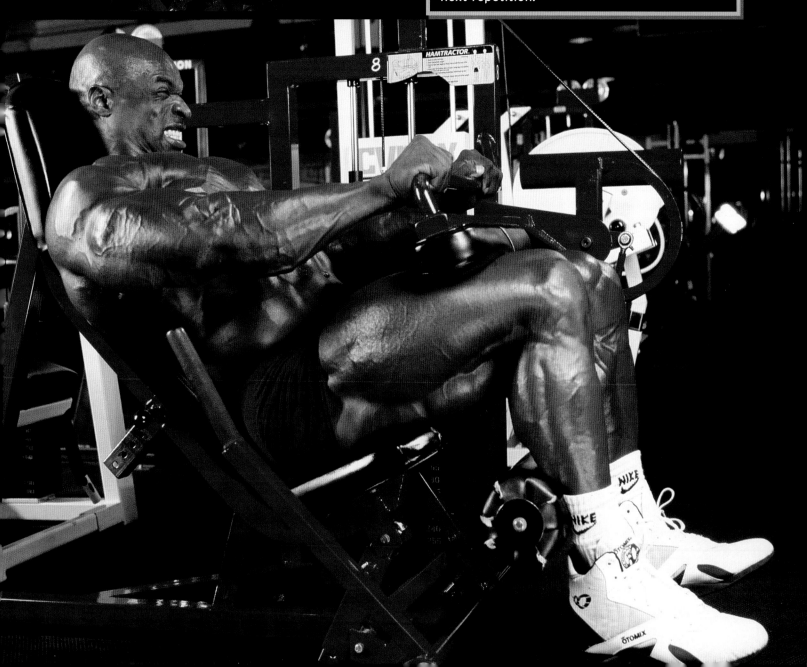

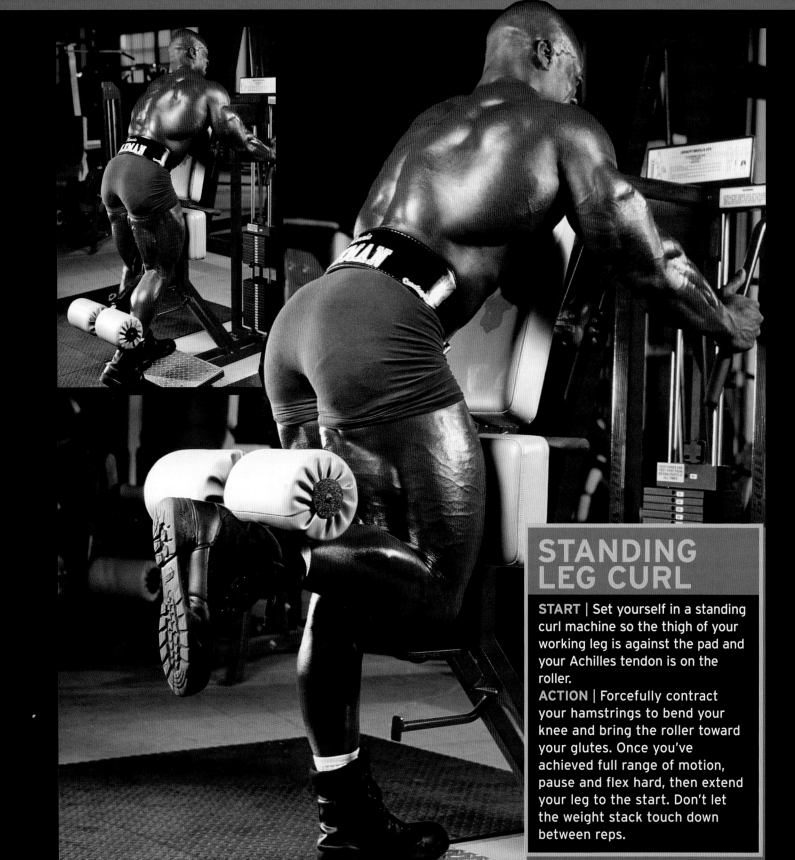

STANDING LEG CURL

START | Set yourself in a standing curl machine so the thigh of your working leg is against the pad and your Achilles tendon is on the roller.

ACTION | Forcefully contract your hamstrings to bend your knee and bring the roller toward your glutes. Once you've achieved full range of motion, pause and flex hard, then extend your leg to the start. Don't let the weight stack touch down between reps.

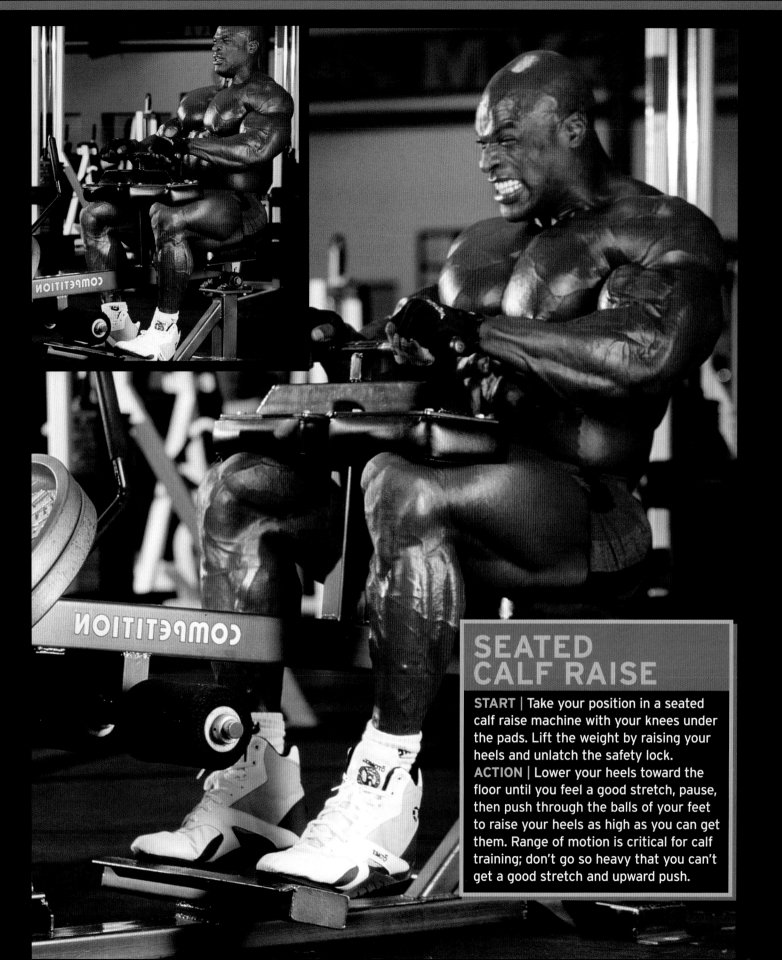

SEATED CALF RAISE

START | Take your position in a seated calf raise machine with your knees under the pads. Lift the weight by raising your heels and unlatch the safety lock.

ACTION | Lower your heels toward the floor until you feel a good stretch, pause, then push through the balls of your feet to raise your heels as high as you can get them. Range of motion is critical for calf training; don't go so heavy that you can't get a good stretch and upward push.

Ronnie's Leg Lessons

1 YOUR QUADS are made up of four separate muscles. Four is better than one when trying to push a heavy load, so the quads are capable of moving a lot of weight. But on the flip side, four muscles also require more attention than one does, and people often have trouble bringing up their quads because of this. If you're having problems, try training them twice a week using different exercises each time to keep the muscles from adapting to one routine.

2 I TRAIN MY QUADS with pretty heavy weights to put on size, but I also keep my rep range high. Because of the sheer amount of stress my legs are under from this type of training, I've been able to develop a level of density in my muscle fibers that a lower rep range wouldn't provide.

3 I USE A LOT OF COMPOUND leg exercises like squats and lunges when I train quads. Yes, they work my hamstrings and glutes as well, but because of that, I can ultimately lift more weight and really attack my quads. Compound exercises also elevate my heart rate during my workout, giving me a little added fat-burning action without a treadmill.

4 IF YOU HAVE BACK PROBLEMS, you can do squats safely if you pay attention to correct form and precise execution. I've had back problems for the last 15 years, and I'm a stickler for form when squatting to avoid aggravating my injuries. If squats annoy your injury no matter what you do, stick to supported exercises like leg presses and hack squats.

5 I SEE A LOT OF PEOPLE doing leg presses one leg at a time, which is fine if all you're going for is detail, but singling out each leg would defeat my purpose for doing them. For me, leg presses are mass-builders, and I push a really heavy weight to develop the most size possible with this exercise. Obviously, you're going to press less weight with one leg than with two, so I train both legs together on this one, and use leg extensions to satisfy my need for detail.

6 USE AN EXPLOSIVE ACTION on the positive contraction of your quadriceps and hamstring exercises. This helps not only to separate and define the muscles but it adds serious size to my legs. You've never seen a sprinter with wimpy quads because they train explosively all the time.

7 NO MATTER WHICH quad exercise you do, never ever lock out your knees. You'll want to come as close as possible to lockout on leg extensions, but even on those, don't extend your legs to the point at which they can go no further (and especially, don't snap them up to the finish, as I've watched some people do). When it comes to leg training, knee lockout equals bad form, and may lead to injuries such as strains, sprains and hyperextensions.

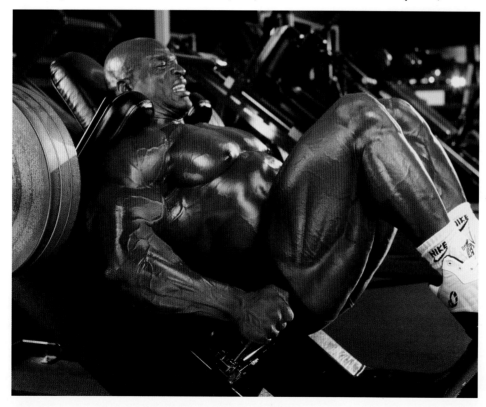

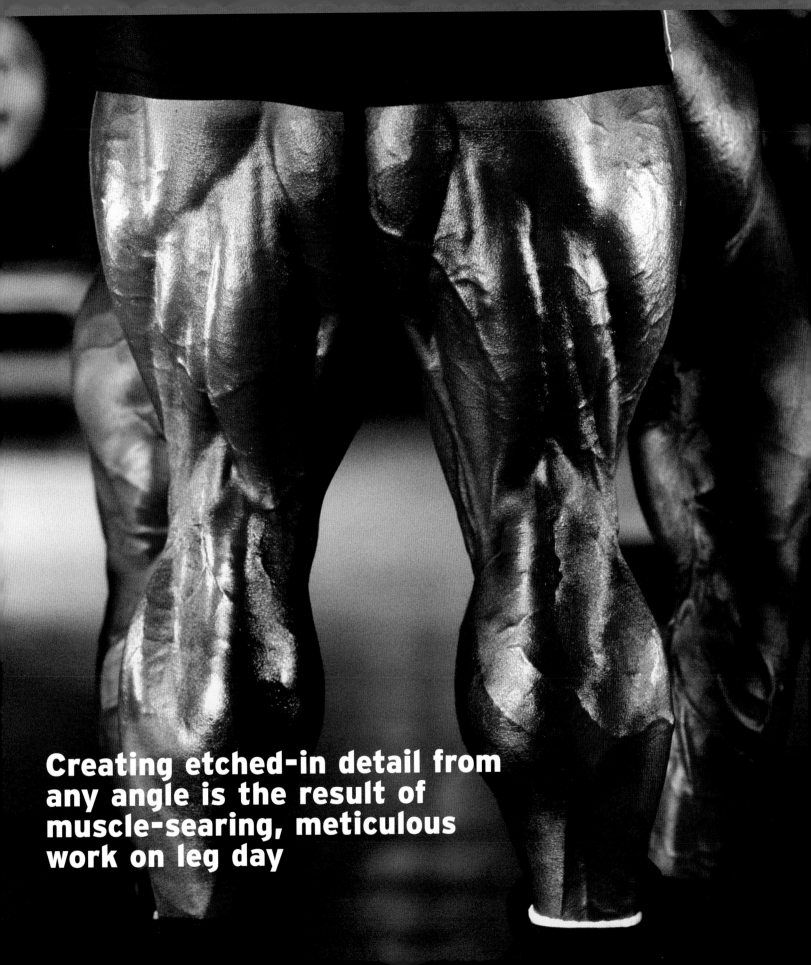

Creating etched-in detail from any angle is the result of muscle-searing, meticulous work on leg day

CHAPTER 5
WIDEN YOUR DELTS

One of the most frequent compliments I receive concerns my exaggerated hourglass shape, an impression created mostly by my big, sweeping back, topped off by a wide shoulder structure and swollen delts. Yet what most people don't realize is that for years, my deltoid development was far behind that of the rest of my body.

When I was a powerlifter, long before I even considered taking up bodybuilding, I was concerned only with building strength, not refining my physique. While my heavy bench presses, deadlifts and squats gave me an exceptionally wide, thick and powerful shoulder girdle, they did not permit my individual deltoid heads to stand out with their own distinct separations from the rest of my shoulder complex. I had more than enough size but no deltoid shape. As a big and muscular guy, I was light-years ahead of the pack. As a bodybuilder, I had to play lots of catch-up.

Obviously, I wasn't going to close the gap merely by hitting my delts heavier. If I expected to bring my delts up to the standard of the rest of my body, I needed to do something creative for them, alone. What I found was a combination of solutions which have proven so successful that I've been using them ever since. By following my workout, I'm sure you can boost your shoulder development, too.

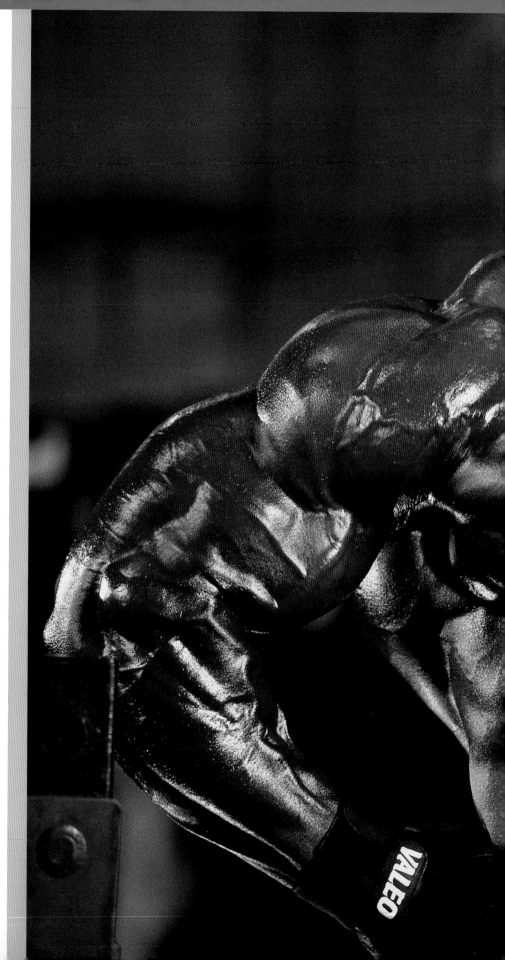

BEGIN WITH A PRESS, either with dumbbells, a barbell or a Smith machine. Start off nice and light — the shoulder joint is delicate, so it's better to go a little overboard on warming up the area by adding an extra set or two of warm-ups. (You can even consider an extremely light set of lateral raises for 25–30 reps). Once you get into the groove, go up in weight from set to set.

Presses attack all three heads of the deltoid muscle, giving a lot of work to the front and middle while also engaging the rear heads to a lesser extent. Once you have the press out of the way, it's time to give a little love to all three heads separately. It doesn't matter which order you do the next three exercises, and you may even want to switch it up from workout to workout. In any case, in the regimen presented here, I pump the side delts first with standing laterals, then move to front raises, and finally to bent-over laterals. While dumbbells are an effective weapon of choice for the shoulder, cables or machines can sometimes be substituted — cables provide constant tension all the way through lateral-type moves, making them a solid part of your shoulder workout rotation.

Try pyramiding up your weights when doing side laterals. After experimenting with this training technique for only two weeks, I found that my shoulders were getting wider, thicker and more impressive. I had smashed that training barrier and was moving on up to the penthouse of bodybuilding success. Here's how I organize my side laterals using the pyramiding training principle: I start with 30-pound dumbbells for 25 reps, 40-pounders for 15, 50-pounders for 12 and 60-pounders for 10. I do this quadruple pyramiding set twice with no rest between each dumbbell switch. I don't use this particular approach on my front delts or rear delts, but that doesn't mean you can't if either of those heads is weak for you.

RONNIE'S DELT WORKOUT

EXERCISE	SETS	REPS
Smith-Machine Seated Press	4	15, 15 12, 10
Dumbbell Lateral Raise	2*	20/15/ 12/10
Dumbbell Front Raise	3	12
Bent-Over Lateral Raise	3	12

*In this reverse-drop set, I'll pyramid up the weights while dropping the reps; do 20 reps, drop the weight, do 15 reps, drop the weight, etc. Don't rest between drops, and run through this four-drop set twice total.

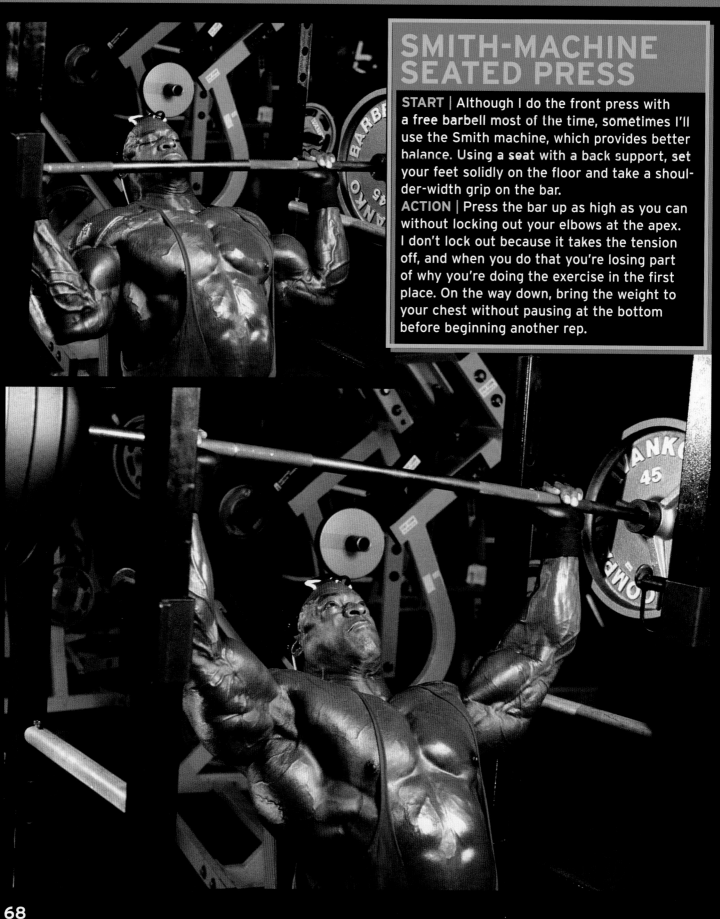

SMITH-MACHINE SEATED PRESS

START | Although I do the front press with a free barbell most of the time, sometimes I'll use the Smith machine, which provides better balance. Using a seat with a back support, set your feet solidly on the floor and take a shoulder-width grip on the bar.

ACTION | Press the bar up as high as you can without locking out your elbows at the apex. I don't lock out because it takes the tension off, and when you do that you're losing part of why you're doing the exercise in the first place. On the way down, bring the weight to your chest without pausing at the bottom before beginning another rep.

DUMBBELL LATERAL RAISE

START | Stand with your feet shoulder-width apart, holding two dumbbells with your palms facing each other, maintaining a slight bend in your elbows so the weights begin in front of your hips. If you prefer, you can also start with the dumbbells at your sides; either way is effective, so it's just a matter of preference.

ACTION | Contract your delts and lead with the weights until they come up and out to your sides. Your upper arms should be parallel with the floor at the top. With only a brief pause at the apex, continue with a slow and controlled movement back to the start position and immediately begin another rep. Sometimes I'll switch up and use cables for a change of pace.

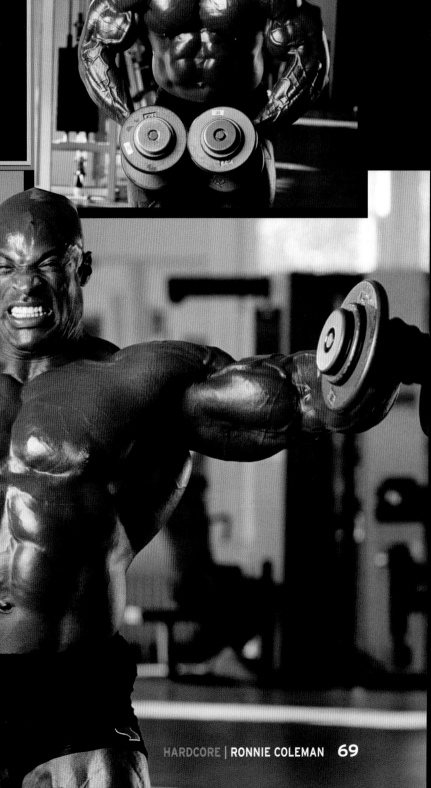

DUMBBELL FRONT RAISE

START | Stand with your feet shoulder-width apart, holding two dumbbells with your palms facing the sides of your thighs and with a slight bend in both of your elbows.

ACTION | Lift one weight in front of yourself to just above level with the top of your head, twisting your wrist so your palm faces the floor at the top. I hold it there for a brief second, then lower the dumbbell back down. After returning to the start position with that first dumbbell, immediately switch arms and follow the same procedure to complete one full rep. On this move, sometimes I'll use a barbell for variety's sake. You can also try the dumbbell version using a palms-facing (hammer) grip the entire time instead of performing the twist on the "up" phase. For efficiency and a change of pace, front raises can be paired with side laterals – do a front raise and a lateral raise with one arm, then the other, alternating until you complete 12 reps of each move per arm.

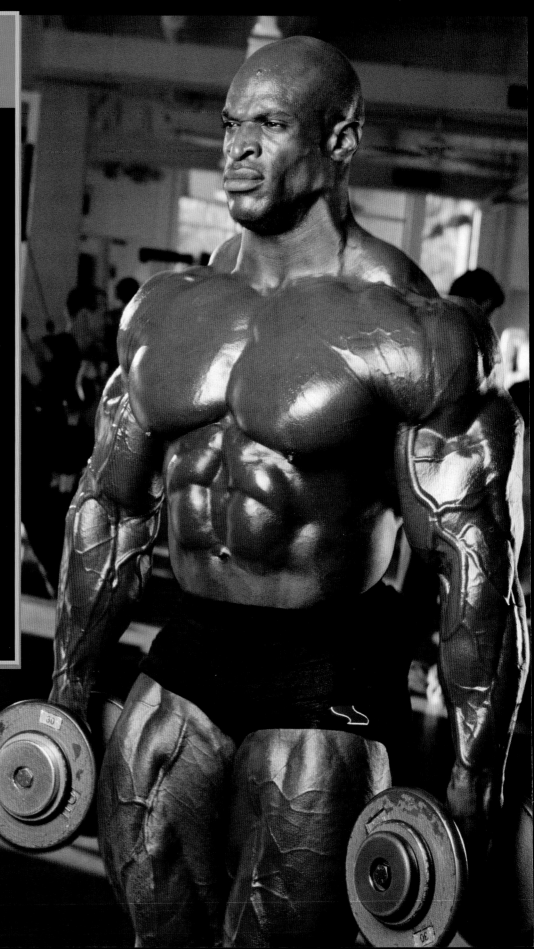

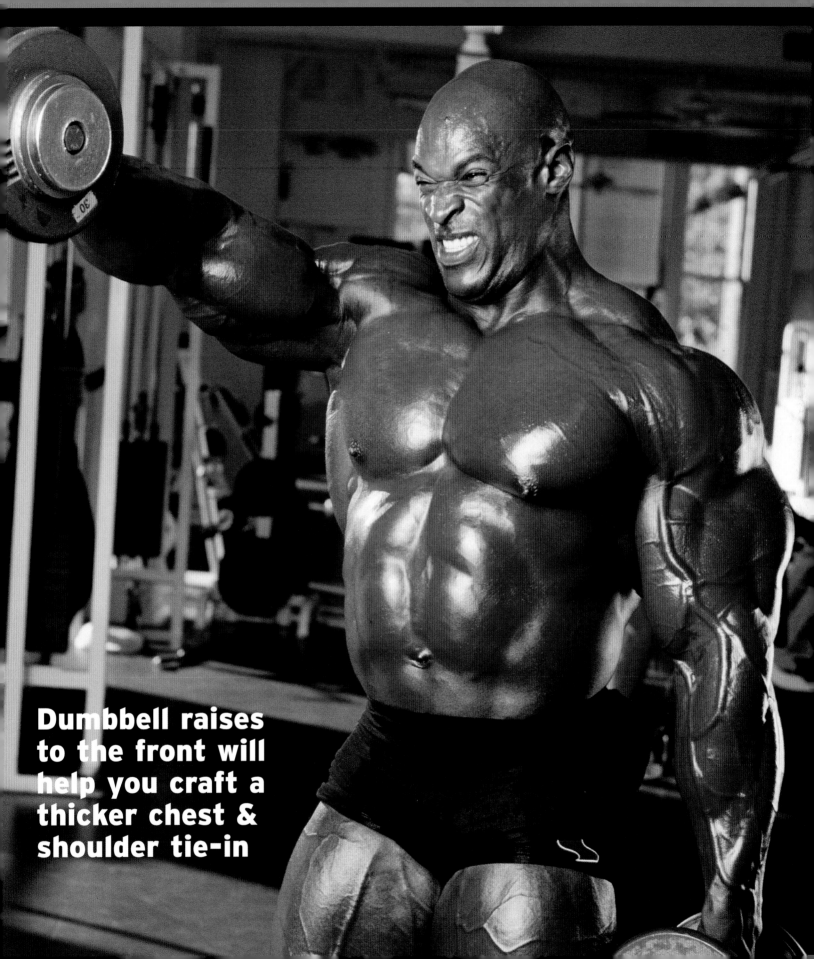

Dumbbell raises to the front will help you craft a thicker chest & shoulder tie-in

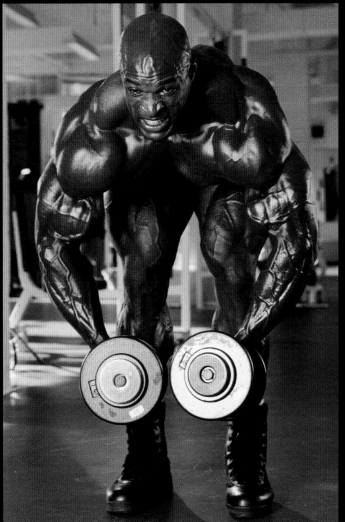

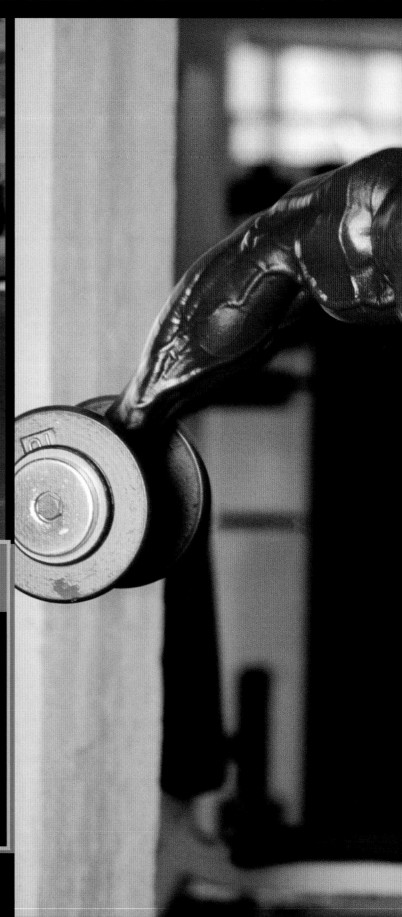

BENT-OVER
LATERAL RAISE

START | Grasp two dumbbells, hold them at your sides and bend your knees slightly. Your feet should be shoulder-width apart and your elbows a bit bent. I try to keep my torso at a 45-degree angle. I look up into the mirror and use a weight that's light enough for me to keep steady. If you find your upper body is bouncing up during execution, you're going too heavy.

ACTION | In a slow and controlled movement, raise the weights out to your sides until your arms are about parallel to the floor. Hold the peak contraction for a second before returning to the start position.

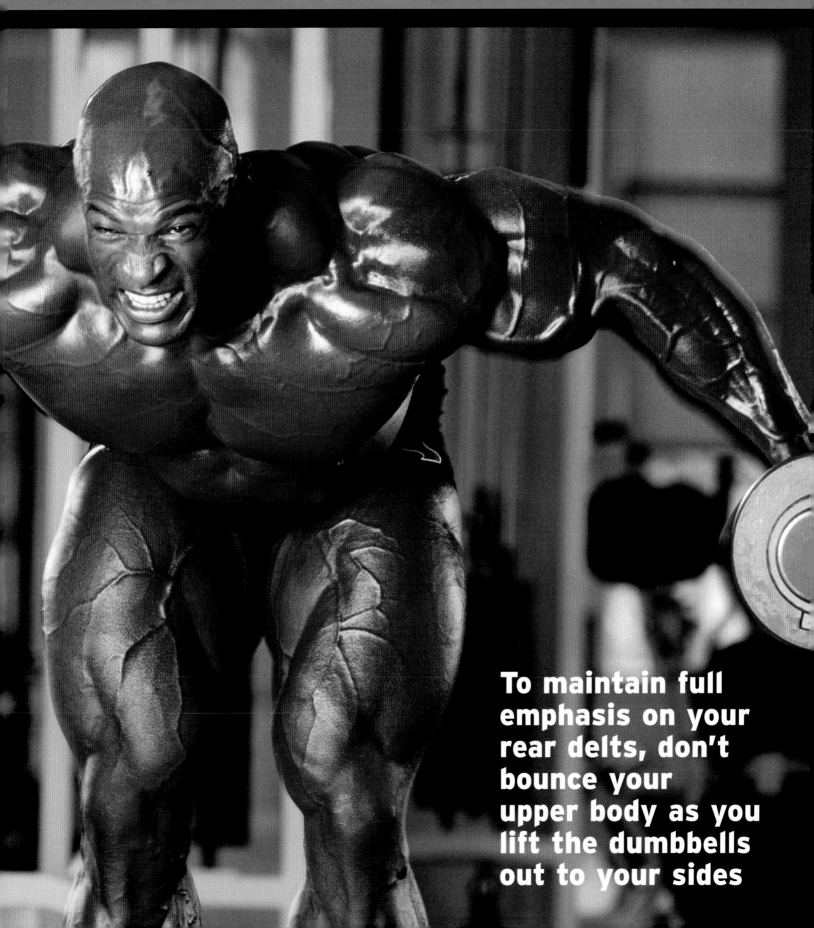

To maintain full emphasis on your rear delts, don't bounce your upper body as you lift the dumbbells out to your sides

Final Notes

A few words of caution: Don't try to keep up with me right off the bat. I've been at this for more than half my life, and it took me that long to get to this level. Don't just go into the gym and start throwing huge poundages around; proceed gradually, making progress in your weights more over months rather than in spikes from workout to workout.

And as always, make each repetition count. When you train deltoids, the objective is to specifically stress hard-to-reach, isolated muscles. To accomplish that, you need to be an expert bodybuilder who possesses all of the maturity and intelligence that term implies. Train your deltoids hard, but train them smart. They'll grow faster.

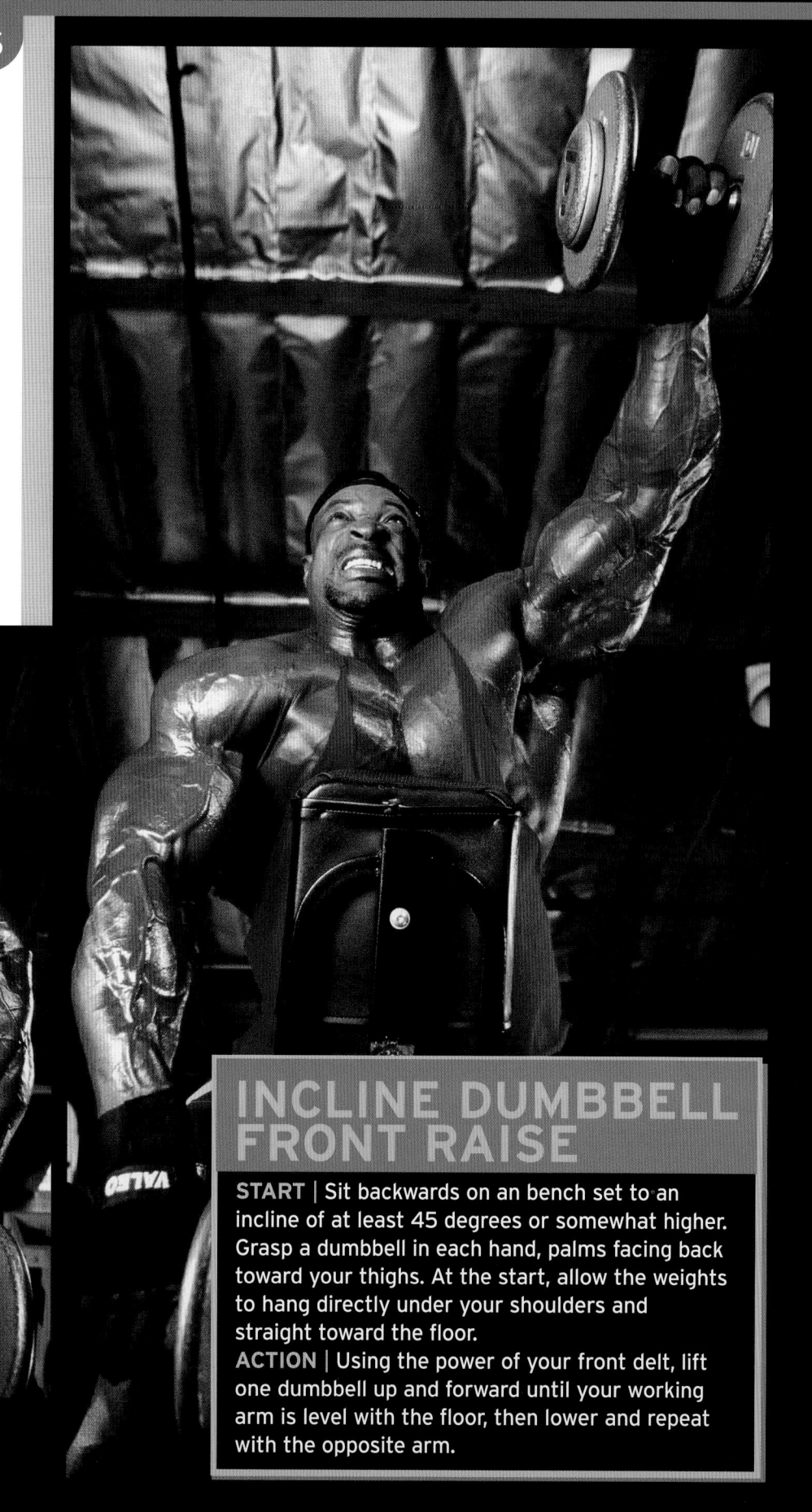

INCLINE DUMBBELL FRONT RAISE

START | Sit backwards on an bench set to an incline of at least 45 degrees or somewhat higher. Grasp a dumbbell in each hand, palms facing back toward your thighs. At the start, allow the weights to hang directly under your shoulders and straight toward the floor.

ACTION | Using the power of your front delt, lift one dumbbell up and forward until your working arm is level with the floor, then lower and repeat with the opposite arm.

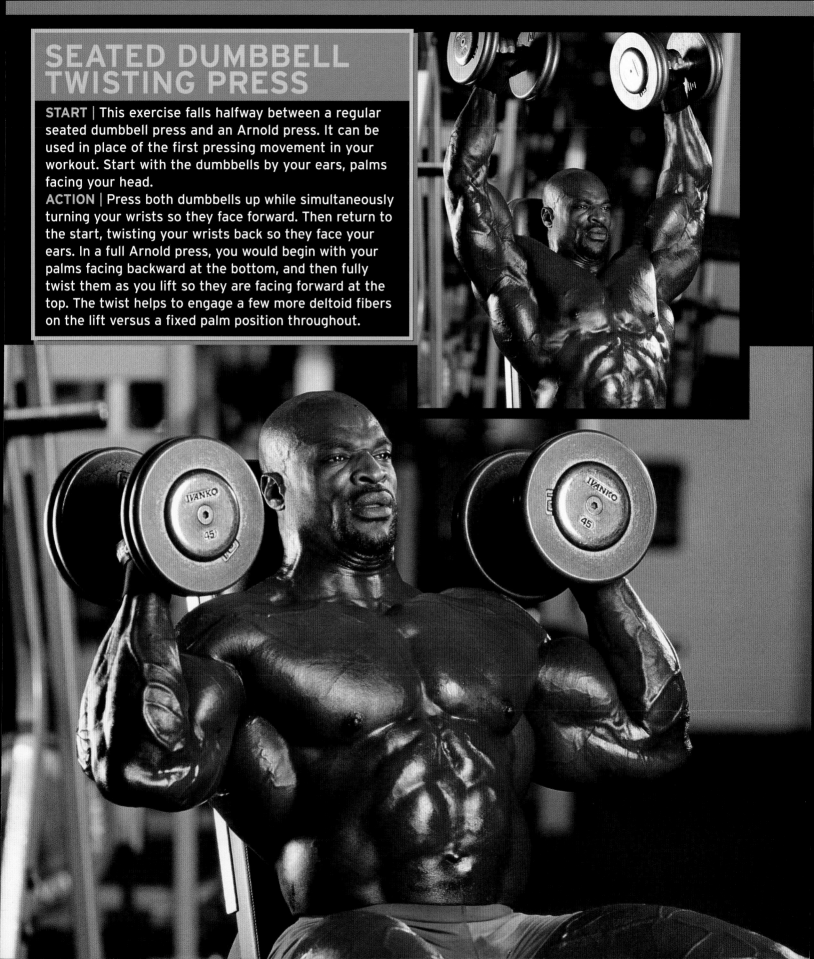

SEATED DUMBBELL TWISTING PRESS

START | This exercise falls halfway between a regular seated dumbbell press and an Arnold press. It can be used in place of the first pressing movement in your workout. Start with the dumbbells by your ears, palms facing your head.

ACTION | Press both dumbbells up while simultaneously turning your wrists so they face forward. Then return to the start, twisting your wrists back so they face your ears. In a full Arnold press, you would begin with your palms facing backward at the bottom, and then fully twist them as you lift so they are facing forward at the top. The twist helps to engage a few more deltoid fibers on the lift versus a fixed palm position throughout.

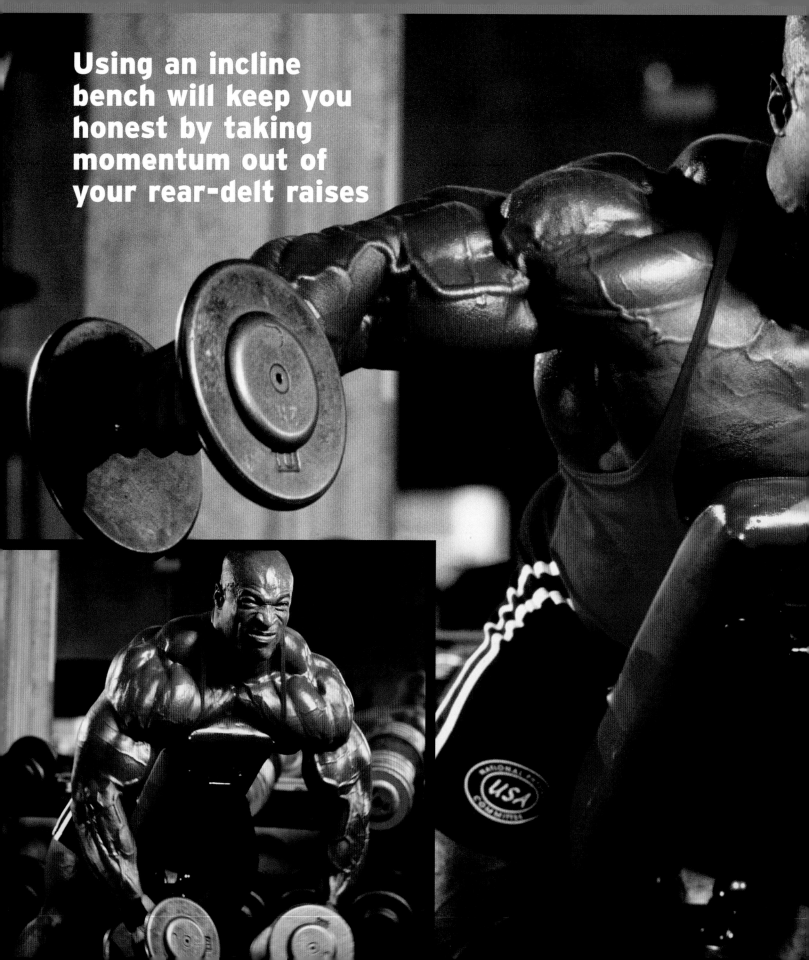

Using an incline bench will keep you honest by taking momentum out of your rear-delt raises

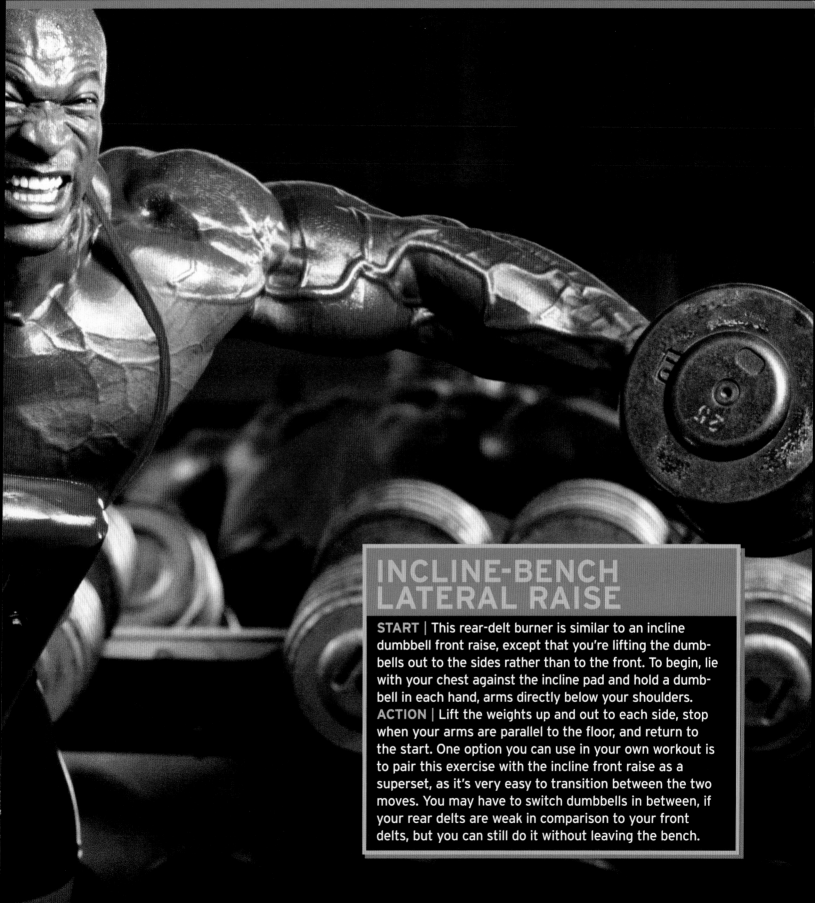

INCLINE-BENCH LATERAL RAISE

START | This rear-delt burner is similar to an incline dumbbell front raise, except that you're lifting the dumb-bells out to the sides rather than to the front. To begin, lie with your chest against the incline pad and hold a dumb-bell in each hand, arms directly below your shoulders.

ACTION | Lift the weights up and out to each side, stop when your arms are parallel to the floor, and return to the start. One option you can use in your own workout is to pair this exercise with the incline front raise as a superset, as it's very easy to transition between the two moves. You may have to switch dumbbells in between, if your rear delts are weak in comparison to your front delts, but you can still do it without leaving the bench.

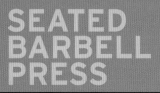

SEATED BARBELL PRESS

START | This strength move separates the men from the boys. Brutally simple, it's all about hoisting a loaded barbell overhead. Start seated on a low-back chair, and grasp a barbell with a grip just outside shoulder width.

ACTION | Generating the power from your delts, lift the barbell straight overhead, stopping just before elbow lockout, then return the barbell to your front clavicles. Throughout, maintain the arch in your lower back and keep your abs tensed for safety.

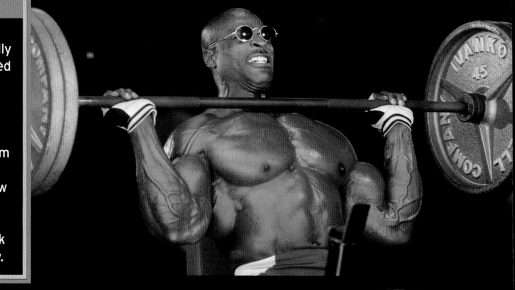

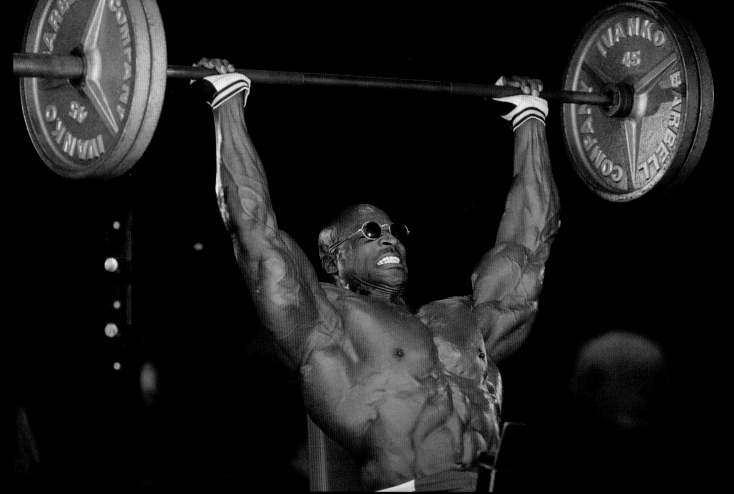

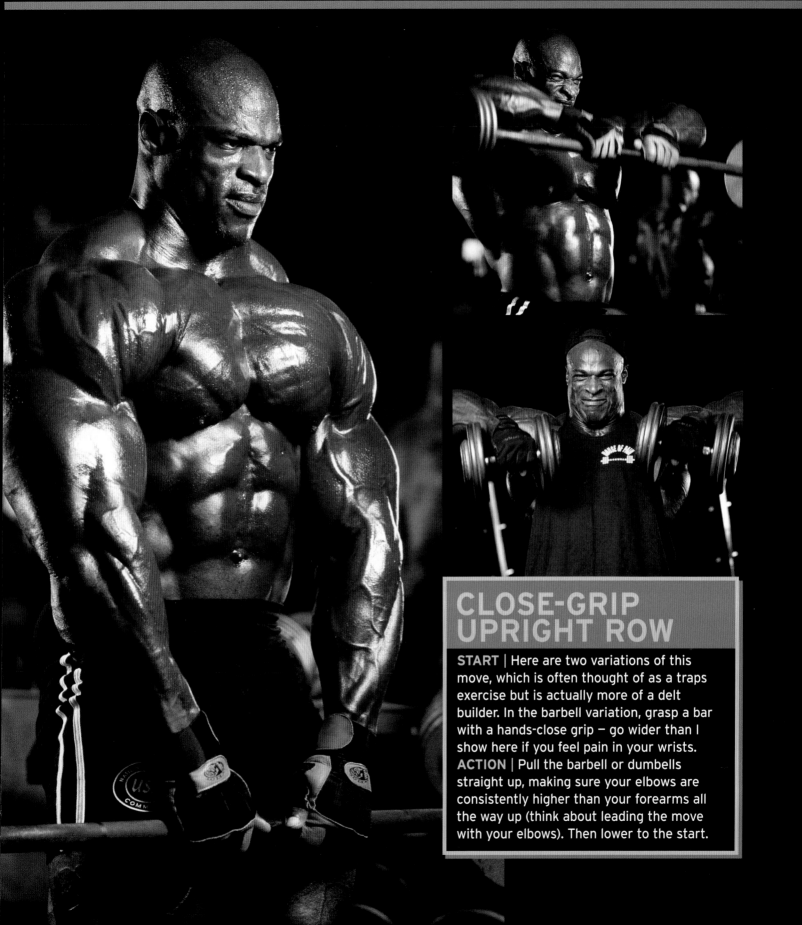

CLOSE-GRIP UPRIGHT ROW

START | Here are two variations of this move, which is often thought of as a traps exercise but is actually more of a delt builder. In the barbell variation, grasp a bar with a hands-close grip – go wider than I show here if you feel pain in your wrists.
ACTION | Pull the barbell or dumbells straight up, making sure your elbows are consistently higher than your forearms all the way up (think about leading the move with your elbows). Then lower to the start.

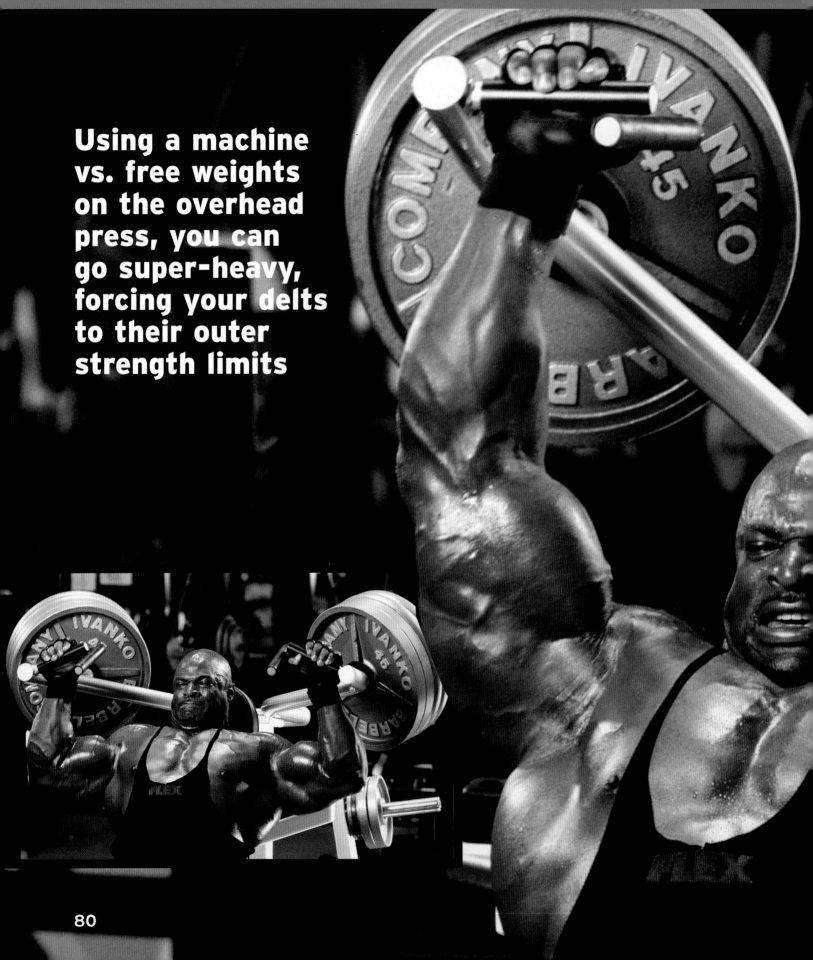

Using a machine vs. free weights on the overhead press, you can go super-heavy, forcing your delts to their outer strength limits

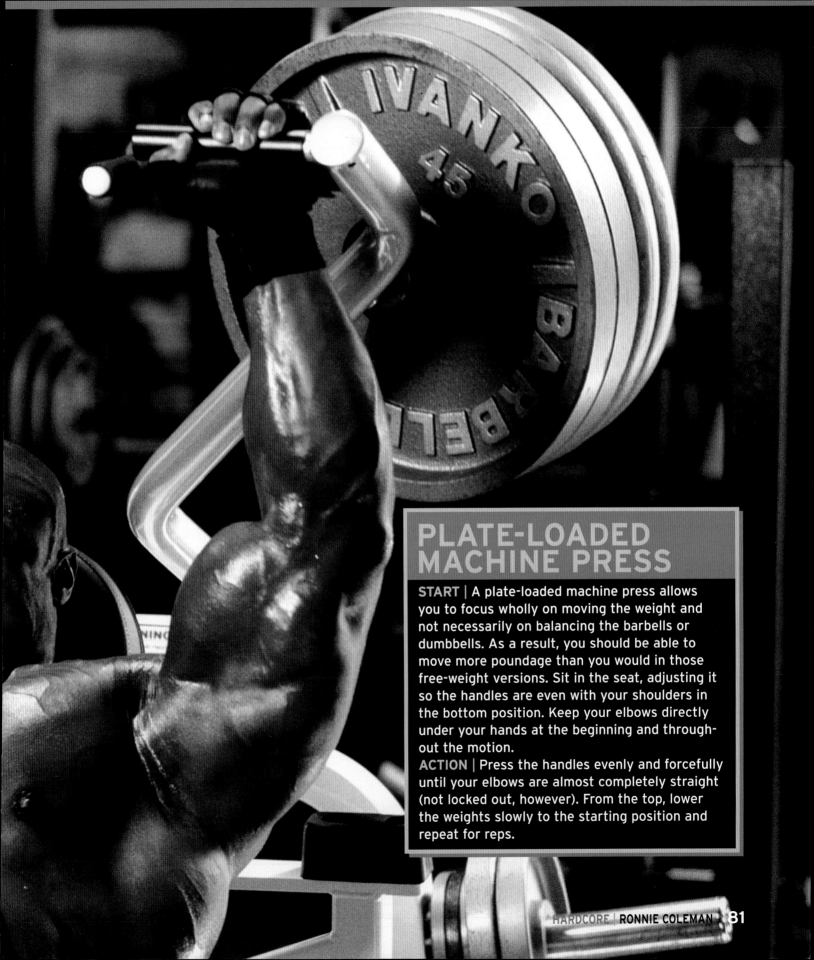

PLATE-LOADED MACHINE PRESS

START | A plate-loaded machine press allows you to focus wholly on moving the weight and not necessarily on balancing the barbells or dumbbells. As a result, you should be able to move more poundage than you would in those free-weight versions. Sit in the seat, adjusting it so the handles are even with your shoulders in the bottom position. Keep your elbows directly under your hands at the beginning and throughout the motion.

ACTION | Press the handles evenly and forcefully until your elbows are almost completely straight (not locked out, however). From the top, lower the weights slowly to the starting position and repeat for reps.

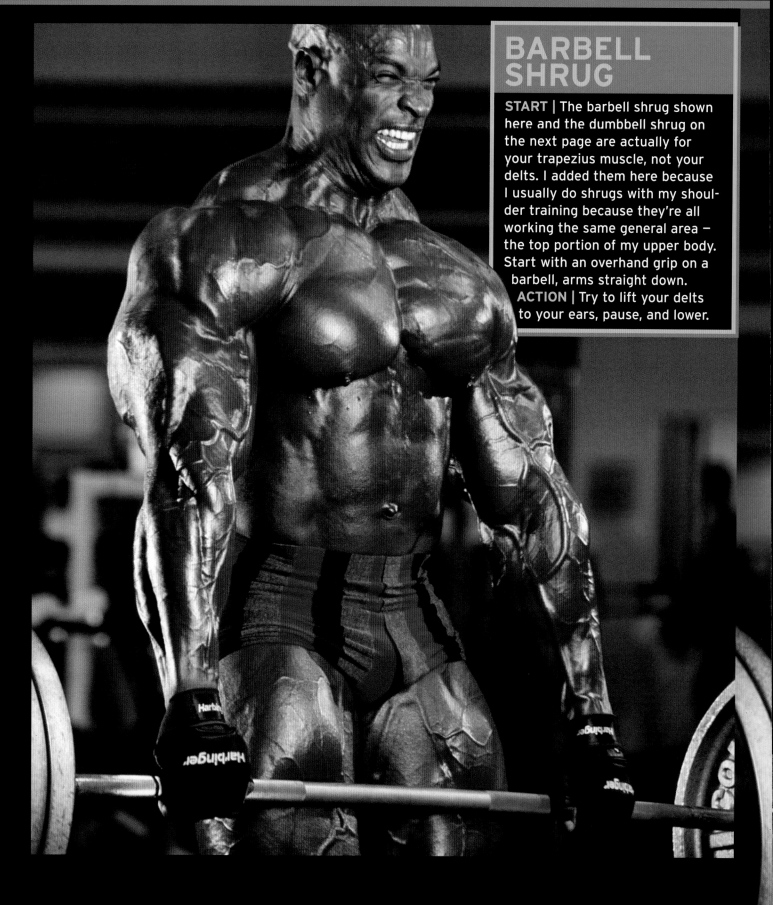

BARBELL SHRUG

START | The barbell shrug shown here and the dumbbell shrug on the next page are actually for your trapezius muscle, not your delts. I added them here because I usually do shrugs with my shoulder training because they're all working the same general area – the top portion of my upper body. Start with an overhand grip on a barbell, arms straight down.
ACTION | Try to lift your delts to your ears, pause, and lower.

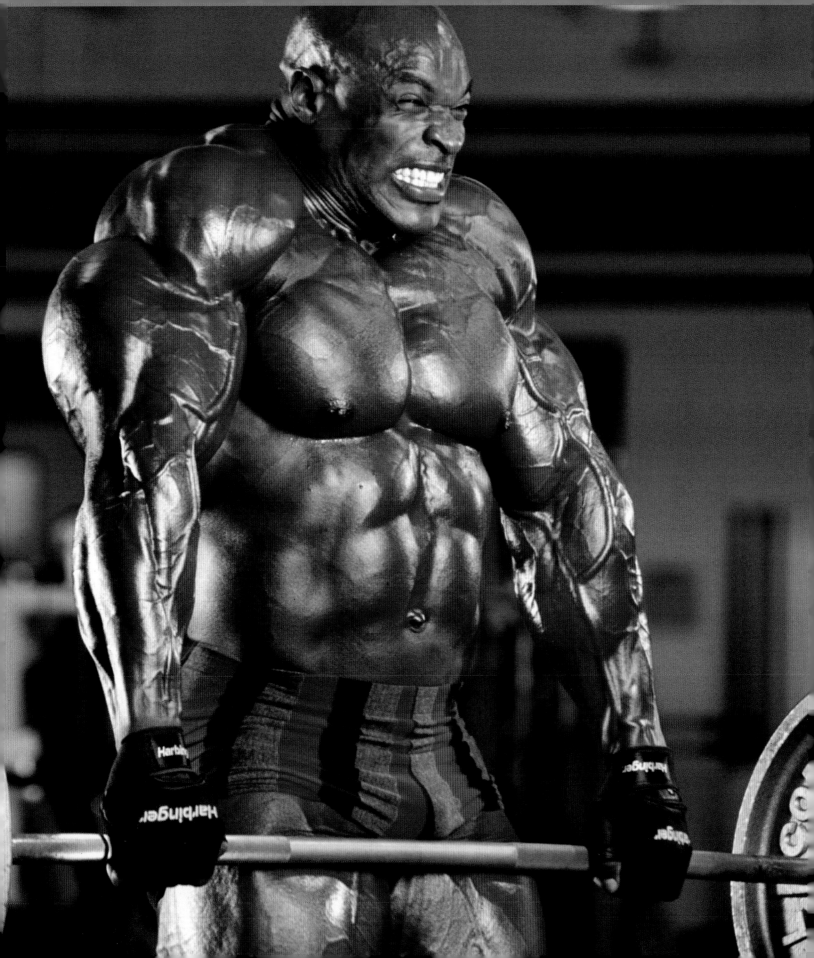

DUMBBELL SHRUG

START | Grasp a pair of dumb-bells at your sides, palms facing in and traps fully stretched. If you feel that it helps, you can use wrist straps to keep your grip, especially on heavy sets because your traps are stronger than your forearms. Otherwise, you may be terminating a set early because your forearms fail while your traps are still strong and ready to go.

ACTION | Forcefully flex your trapezius to shrug your shoulders upward as high as you can. Think about actually trying to touch your delt caps to your ears — you won't be able to physically do it, of course, but going into this move with that thought in mind will assist in pushing you to do full instead of partial reps.

On this exercise and on barbell shrugs (shown on the preceding page), don't bend your elbows as you lift the weights. Some people let their arms get involved in the movement instead of letting the exercise happen completely within the traps (usually when going heavier than they can truly handle), and this cheats you out of valuable development in the area you're trying to target. Save the heavy arm training for your biceps and triceps workouts!

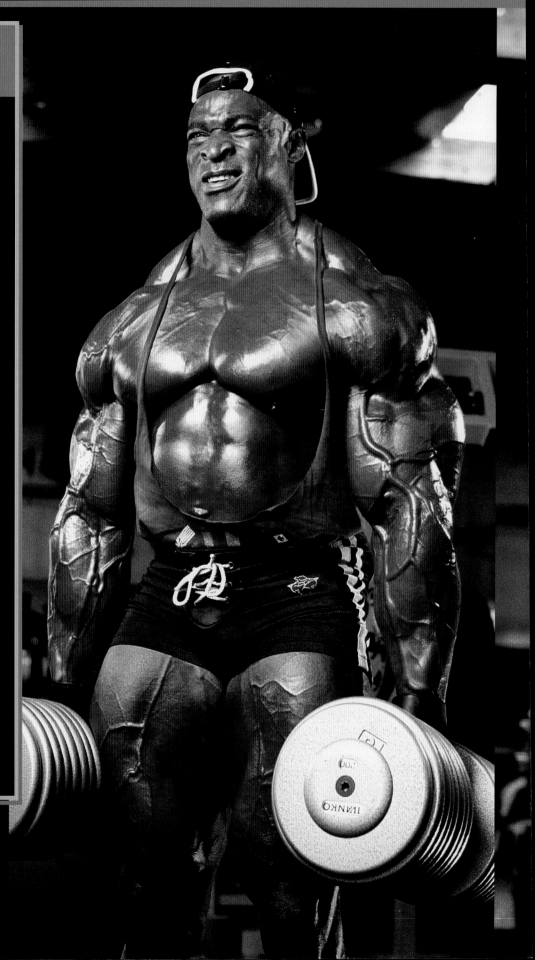

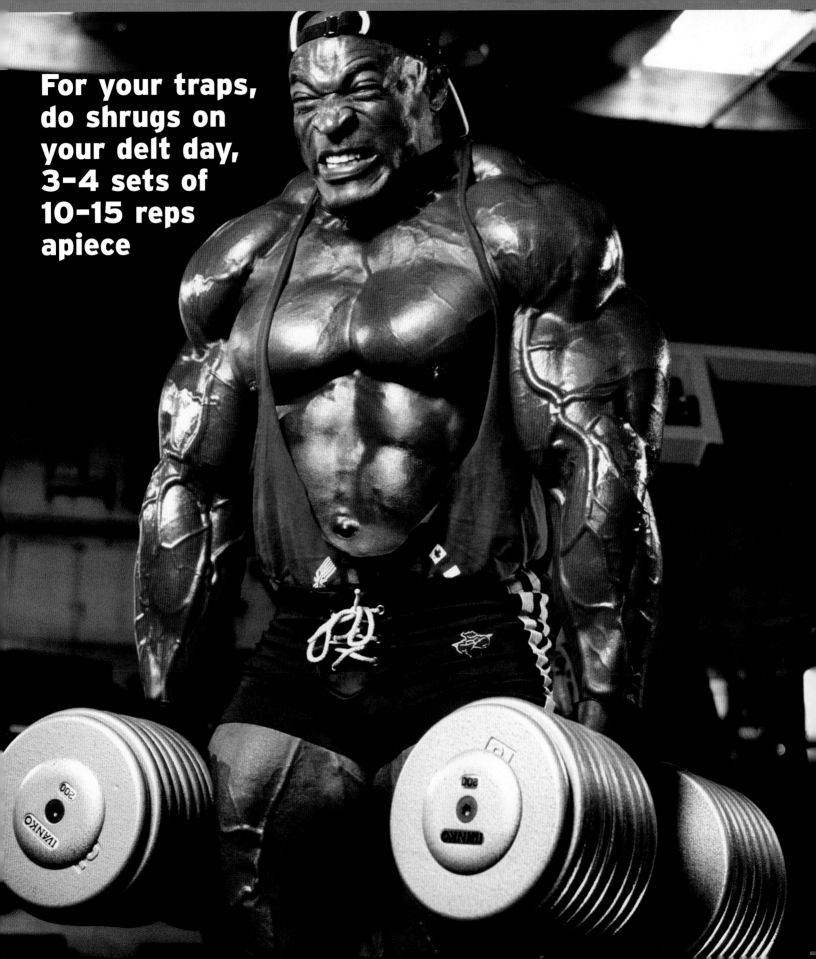

For your traps,
do shrugs on
your delt day,
3-4 sets of
10-15 reps
apiece

Ronnie's Delt Lessons

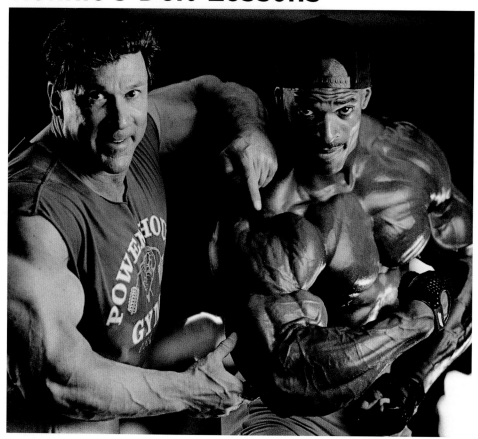

1 THERE'S NO POINT IN DOING a bunch of sets and reps without understanding how the shoulder complex functions. When hitting shoulders, don't think about working a single muscle. Instead, focus on conquering the front, side and rear delts, all of which need focused attention to complete the overall shoulder look you want.

2 MY VERY FIRST SHOULDER PROGRAM consisted of only two exercises: dumbbell shoulder presses and dumbbell lateral raises. Pressing movements are the meat-packing side of the delt-building equation. Presses hit all three heads of the delt triad and build the thickness we all desire. Dumbbell side laterals develop the side delts. Those bad boys help create the illusion of wide shoulders which, when augmented by a narrow waist, seals the deal on a showstopping V-taper.

3 BALANCE IS THE KEY to everything in the sport of bodybuilding, and in building a great body in general. You need to build a well-proportioned physique. No bodypart is more important than another. In the wacky world of delt training, the search for the holy grail of ideal proportions dictates traps and rear delts that can hold their own with front and side delts. That's why you should include rear laterals and shrugs in your comprehensive shoulder-and-trap workout.

4 THE SHOULDER JOINTS are danger zones for bodybuilding injuries. Even if you use correct form doing the exercises I recommend, you'll still risk injury if you lift too heavy. That's why I recommend a two-set, 15-rep warm-up of presses before moving to heavy weights.

5 ALL OF YOUR SHOULDER WORKOUTS should begin with a pressing movement. Shoulder presses are meat-and-potatoes mass builders for front and side delts. They're most effective when your muscles are fresh and ready to rock 'n' roll. After that, I move into the exercises that target each head individually, so no part of my delt escapes a thorough thrashing.

6 RECOVERY TIME makes a big-time difference in your overall results. Generally, I like to train most of my bodyparts twice a week. If your shoulders are a lagging bodypart, you can try to do the same, but you may also want to see what happens when you back it down to once per week. If they start responding, it indicates that you're overtraining and under-recovering.

7 I BELIEVE IN DOING EVERY EXERCISE strictly, so pay close attention to the technique instruction I give in this chapter. Follow my lead carefully and you'll build Texas-size delts that are wide and extremely impressive.

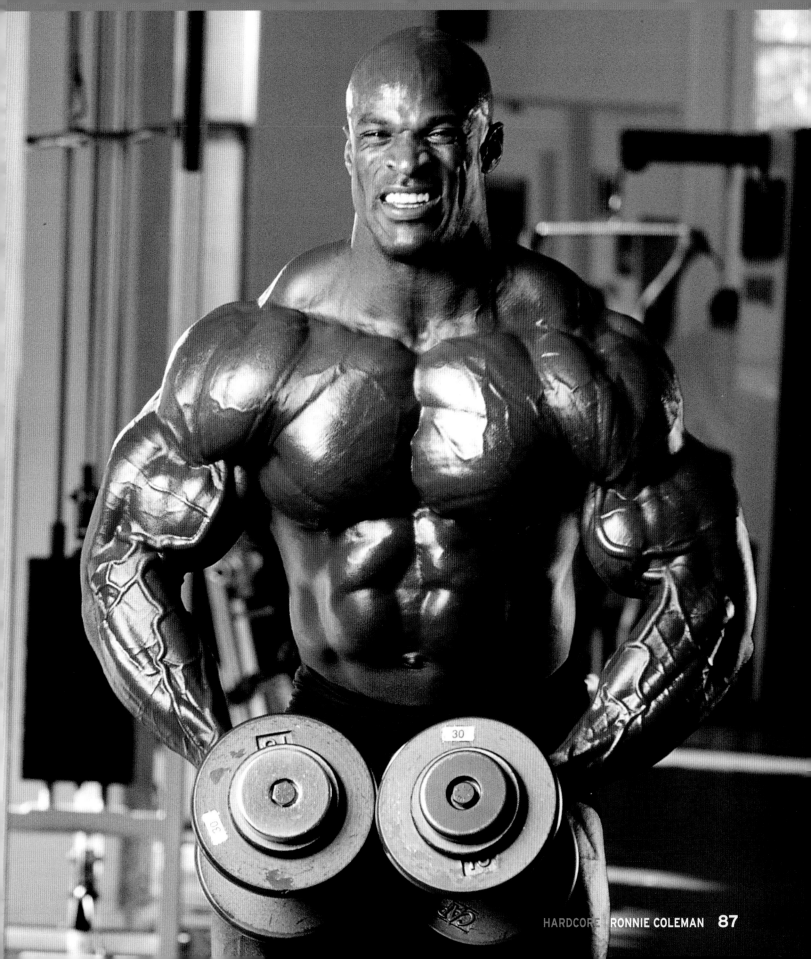

CHAPTER 6
BOMB YOUR BICEPS

Man, my biceps keep growing. That's a mixed blessing. Sure, they've helped me win the Mr. Olympia six times and counting. But on the other hand, I know what it took to build them to this level, and that means I'm in for even more of the same. I'm talking about work – old-fashioned heavy lifting.

Before I started bodybuilding, I had already developed a lot of strength from powerlifting, so when I launched into tons of barbell curls, my biceps exploded. Eventually, though, I noticed that even though my biceps were bowling-ball big, they lacked separations. I didn't even know that these muscles had different names. I couldn't distinguish my biceps brachii from my brachialis. To me, it was all just an arm. That's when I realized I needed to train my biceps with other exercises to bring out additional muscularity.

The results of my current regimen speak for themselves. I get in two biceps workouts a week, and each workout consists of 3-4 exercises, such as the sample ones in this chapter. Something changes in every workout, but it's random. Sometimes, all four exercises will be different; at other times, maybe only one or two will change. But in the end, variety and consistency equal progress.

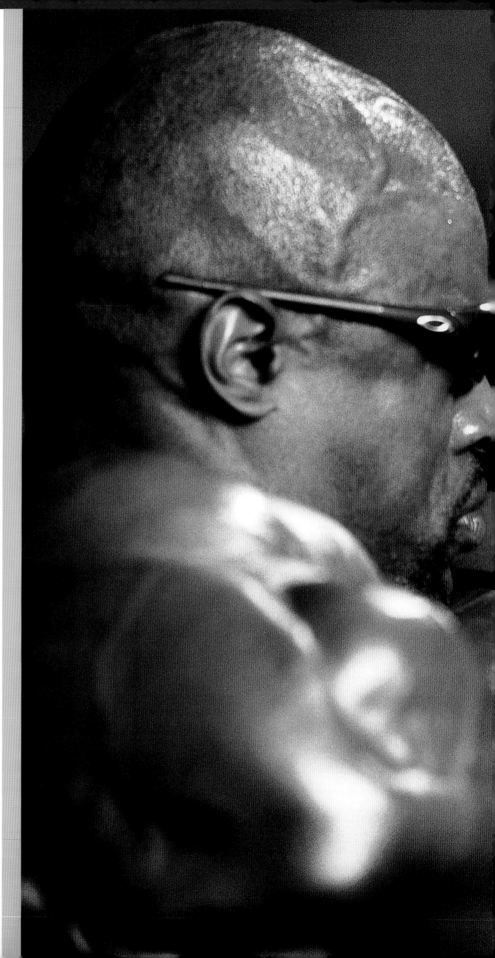

THE ALTERNATING DUMB-
BELL CURL LEADS OFF.
This is one of my favorite
overall mass builders. You can
do these sitting down because
that reduces your ability to use body
english, but I use this is a power
exercise because standing allows me to
use as much weight as I possibly can.
That's not to say that it allows me to
cheat — I never simply swing the weight
— but I can use my balance and power
in unison. Throughout the curl, I focus
on keeping the dumbbell in the same
plane of movement, avoiding any
sideways shifting. I allow my elbows to
come up a little bit at the top, but I try
to keep them fairly close to my side. The
second I complete that rep, I switch my
focus to the opposite arm and begin the
rep on that side. This way, one arm is in
motion at all times, and my focus is
always 100% on the working muscle.

Moving on, I go to the EZ-bar
preacher curl, which works the lower
portion of the biceps. It's really important to allow your biceps to stretch at
the bottom to the point to just before
your elbows reach complete lockout.
This forces the lower part of the muscle
to engage and fire on that initial pull
back up.

The one-arm curl, a cable exercise, is
next. A lot of guys use cables as a burn-
out to exhaust their muscles once and
for all, but I never do that. I treat cables
like any other exercise, going hard and
heavy just as I do with free weights to
make the most of my time in the gym.

I finish up the workout with
dumbbell concentration curls. I don't
see a lot of guys doing this exercise
anymore, but it's one of the best for
crafting thickness throughout the
biceps, as well as developing ample
strength and detail in the forearms.
I like to focus on initiating the motion
from my wrist at the bottom to give
my forearms a little extra action.

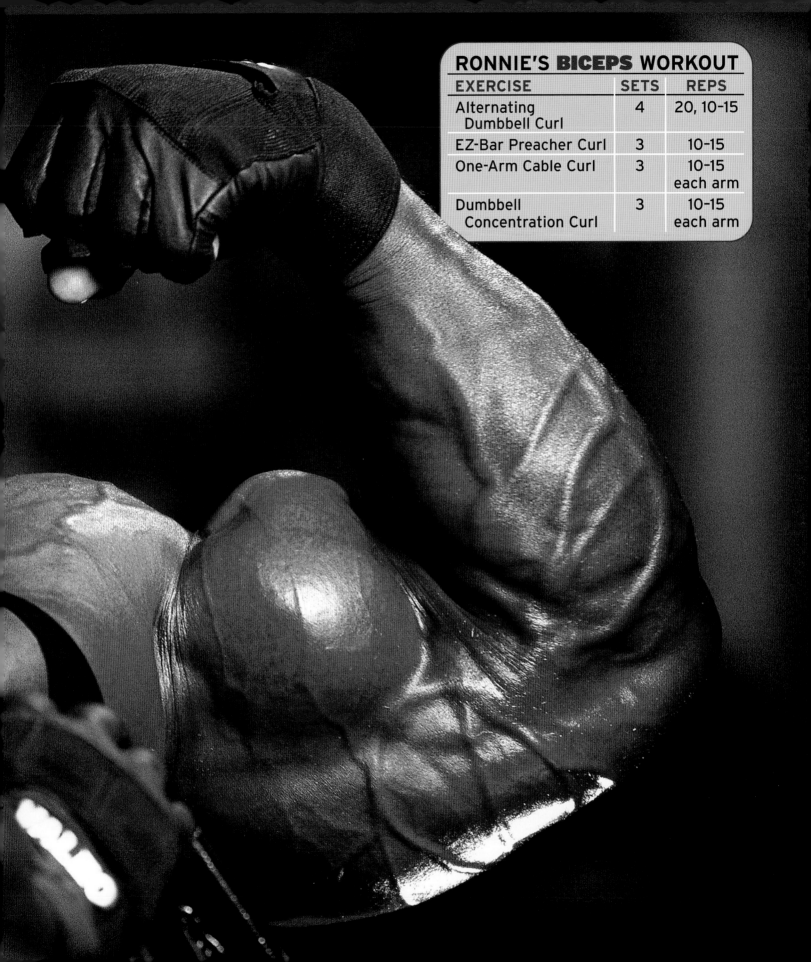

RONNIE'S **BICEPS** WORKOUT

EXERCISE	SETS	REPS
Alternating Dumbbell Curl	4	20, 10-15
EZ-Bar Preacher Curl	3	10-15
One-Arm Cable Curl	3	10-15 each arm
Dumbbell Concentration Curl	3	10-15 each arm

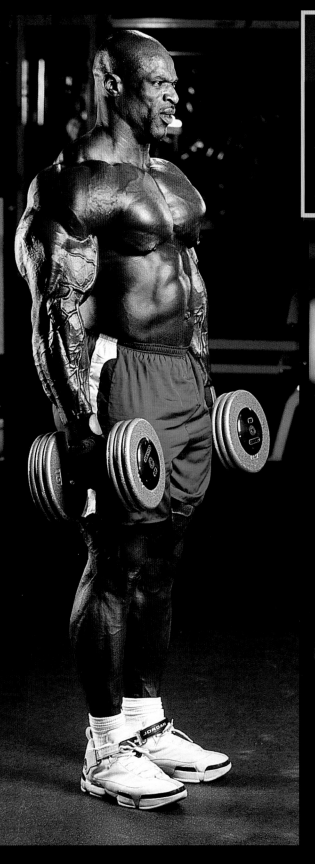

ALTERNATING DUMBBELL CURL

START | Holding a pair of dumbbells at your sides with your palms facing in, stand with your knees slightly bent and your back straight.

ACTION | Using one arm at a time, slowly curl one dumbbell up toward your shoulder, keeping your elbow in and your torso steady to avoid using momentum. Lower, then lift the other dumbbell to complete one full rep.

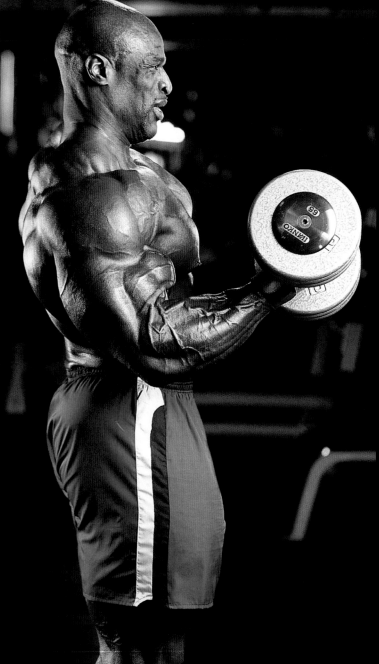

EZ-BAR PREACHER CURL

START | Adjust a preacher bench so the pad comes to a level just under your armpits, and hold an EZ-curl bar on the innermost grips (your palms and wrists will be tilted slightly inward).

ACTION | Starting at the top, slowly lower the bar down toward the pad until your arms are fully extended (but not locked out) and your forearms are flat on the pad. Initiate the upward motion from your wrist and slowly curl the weight toward your delts, squeezing through the peak of your biceps at the top before going onto your next rep.

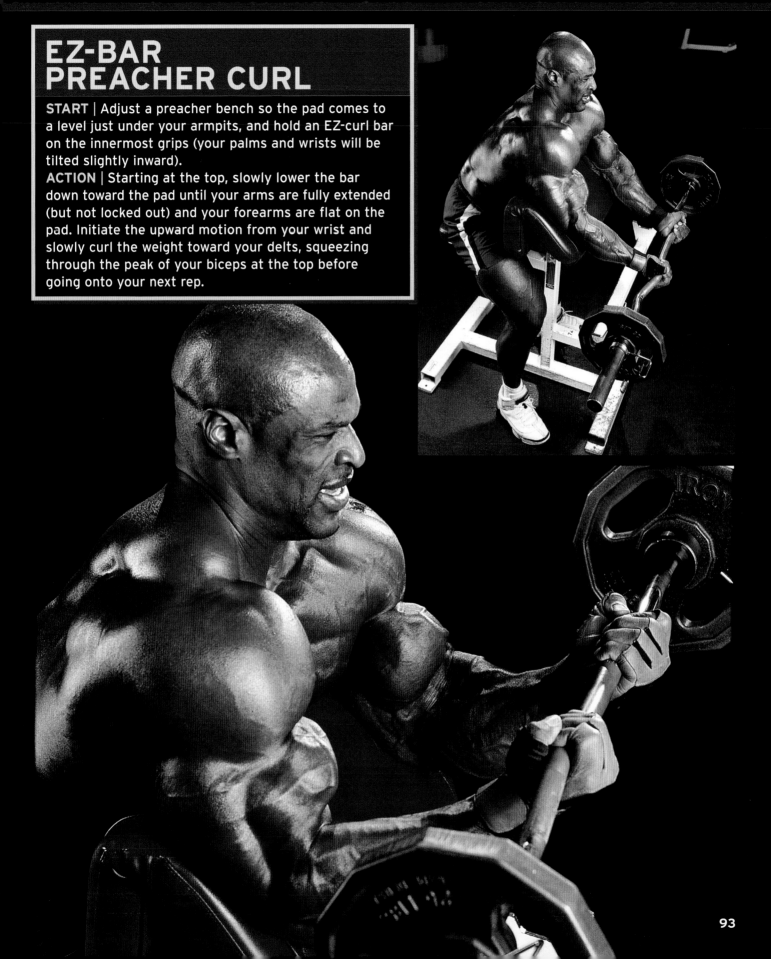

ONE-ARM CABLE CURL

START | Stand facing a cable machine and hold a D-handle attachment in one hand. Bring your working arm slightly to the front of your body and tuck your elbow into your side. Place your opposite hand either on your hip or on the machine for balance.

ACTION | Smoothly curl the handle upward until you reach the point at which you feel your arm might relax. Stop here and squeeze hard through your biceps for a count of two before slowly lowering the handle back to the start, resisting the pull of the cable on the return.

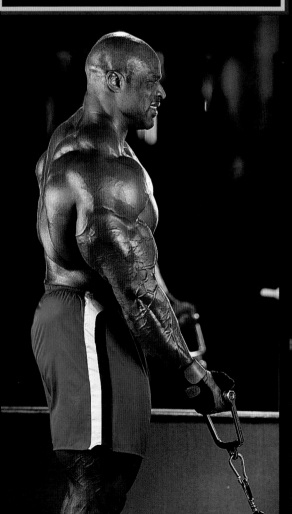
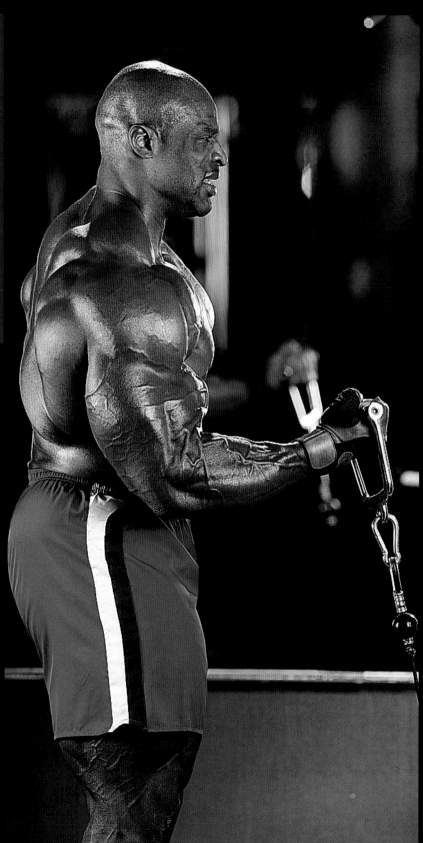

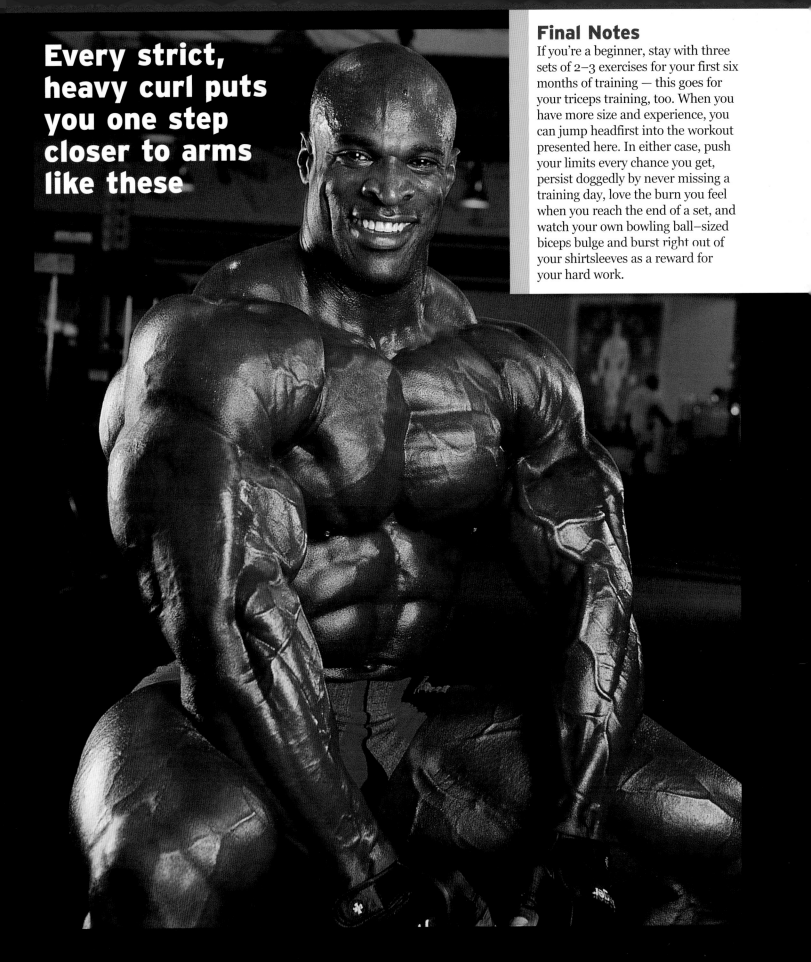

Every strict, heavy curl puts you one step closer to arms like these

Final Notes

If you're a beginner, stay with three sets of 2–3 exercises for your first six months of training — this goes for your triceps training, too. When you have more size and experience, you can jump headfirst into the workout presented here. In either case, push your limits every chance you get, persist doggedly by never missing a training day, love the burn you feel when you reach the end of a set, and watch your own bowling ball–sized biceps bulge and burst right out of your shirtsleeves as a reward for your hard work.

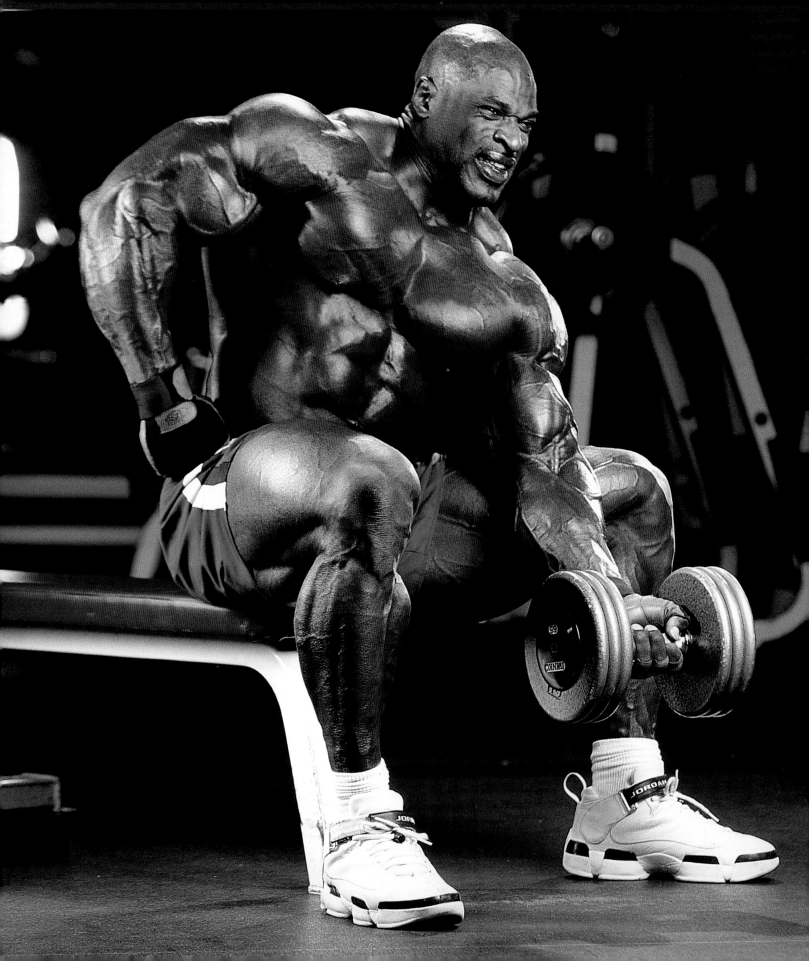

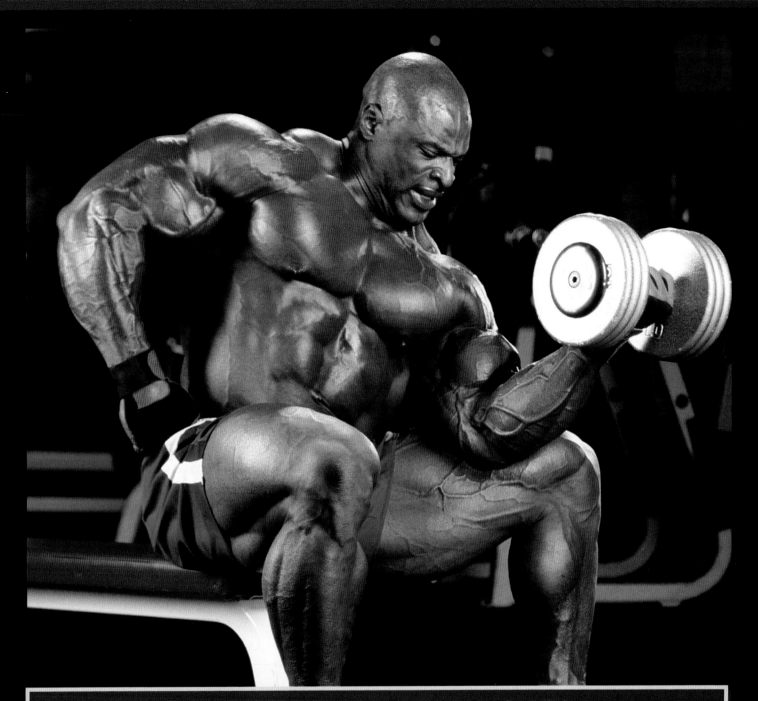

DUMBBELL CONCENTRATION CURL

START | Position yourself at the edge of a bench, grasping a dumbbell in one hand, palm facing upward. Place the elbow of your working arm against the inner portion of your thigh, and put your other hand either on your hip as shown here or in another comfortable location. Keep your head up and maintain the arch in your lower back.

ACTION | Curl the dumbbell toward your shoulder, squeezing it so hard you can almost feel your veins pop through your skin, then lower it back to the start. To protect your elbow joint from hyperextension and to keep tension on the biceps, stop the descent of the dumbbell right before your arm goes completely straight, then go right into the next rep.

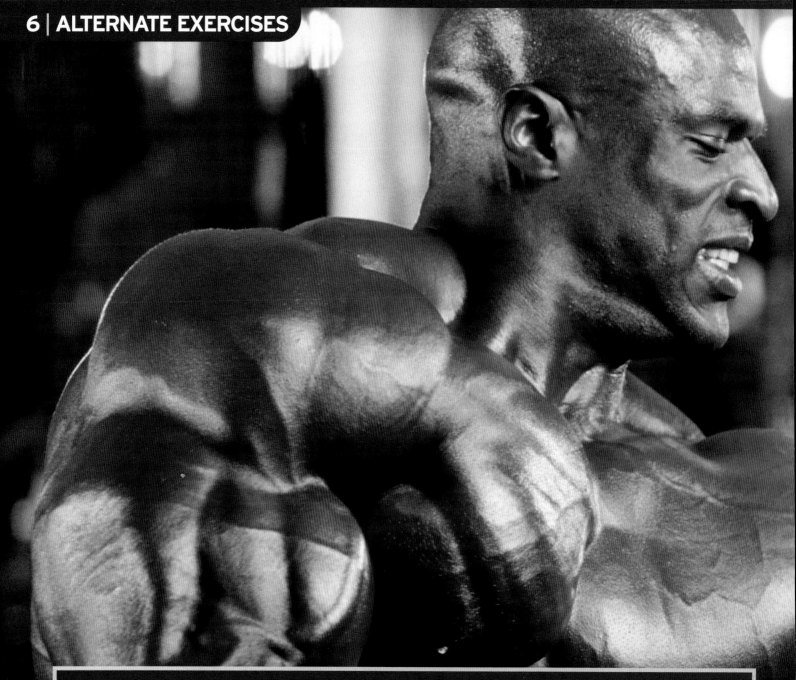

DUMBBELL PREACHER CURL

START | Place your upper arm on the pad – your armpit resting on the peak of the bench – and settle your weight down in a comfortable position. This allows for little movement in the rest of your body, which means you're forced to use all biceps to move the weight. As a result, this is an excellent exercise to achieve almost total isolation. Start with your arm straight (but don't lock out the elbow joint).

ACTION | In a relatively explosive movement, curl the weight up. You should feel a strong and deep contraction in the belly of the working biceps. After finishing your reps for one arm, immediately switch the dumbbell to the opposite hand and do the other side. You only need to take a very short break between sets, because that first arm gets to rest while you complete the reps for the other arm.

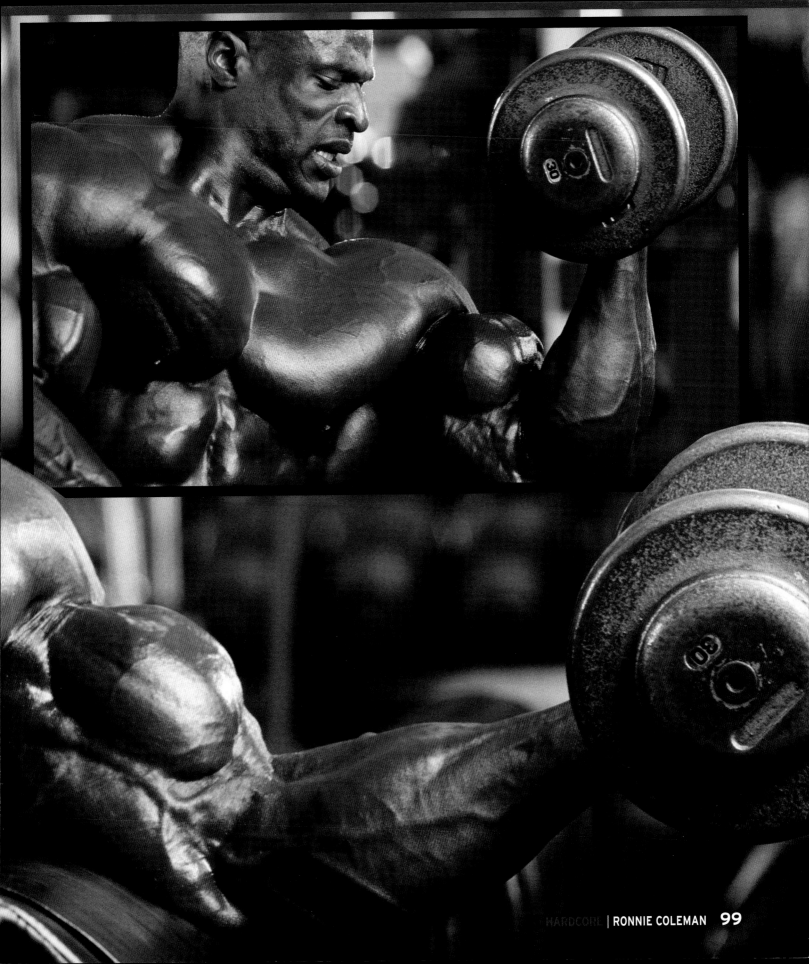

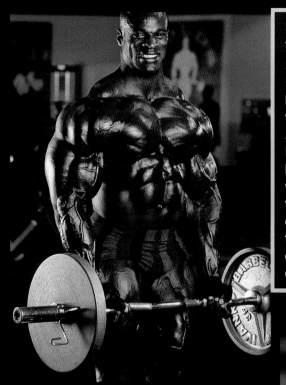

STANDING EZ-BAR CURL

START | This is one of the best mass movements for biceps that I do. I sometimes prefer the EZ-bar to a barbell because it puts less stress on my wrists. I grasp the bar on the outer curls for this exercise, arms almost fully extended.

ACTION | Bring the weight up using only the power of your biceps. Don't swing your body to provide momentum, and concentrate on keeping your elbows by your sides, which forces your biceps to work harder. Forcefully squeeze your biceps at the top, then control the descent; it's easy just to let the weight fall without any controlled resistance, but you lose the benefit of the negative in that case and put yourself at risk for a muscle tear. Concentrate on lowering the weight slowly, taking about twice as long on the downward motion as you do on the positive phase of the rep.

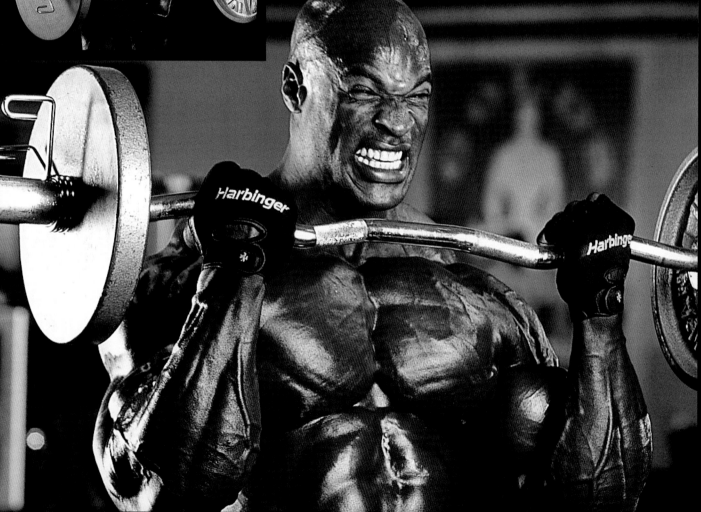

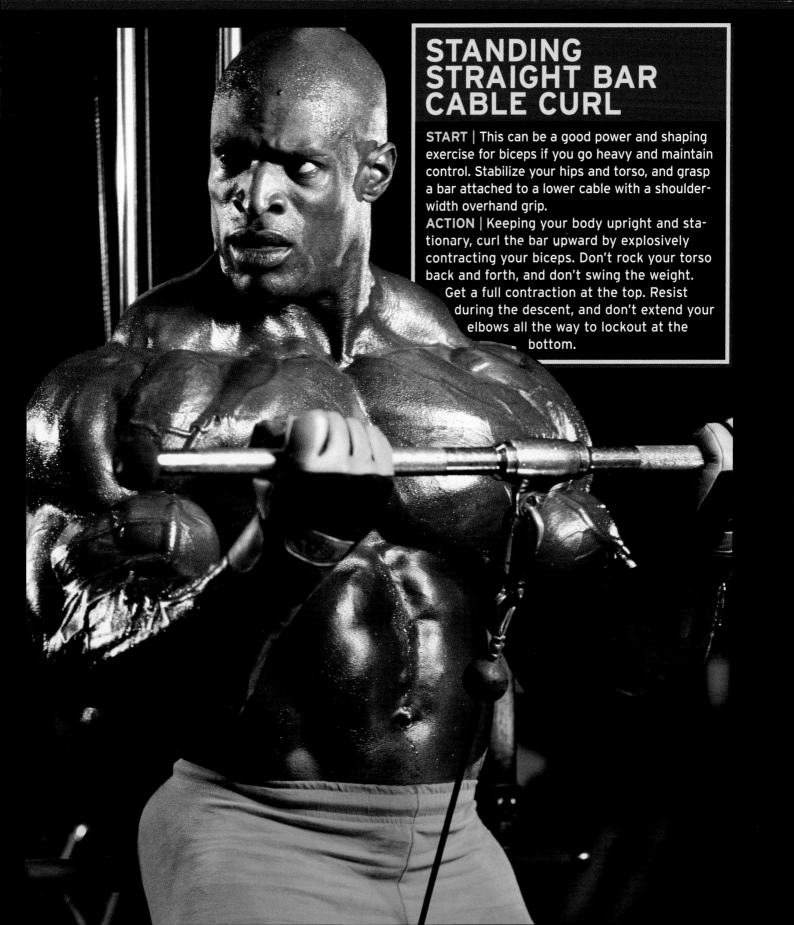

STANDING STRAIGHT BAR CABLE CURL

START | This can be a good power and shaping exercise for biceps if you go heavy and maintain control. Stabilize your hips and torso, and grasp a bar attached to a lower cable with a shoulder-width overhand grip.

ACTION | Keeping your body upright and stationary, curl the bar upward by explosively contracting your biceps. Don't rock your torso back and forth, and don't swing the weight. Get a full contraction at the top. Resist during the descent, and don't extend your elbows all the way to lockout at the bottom.

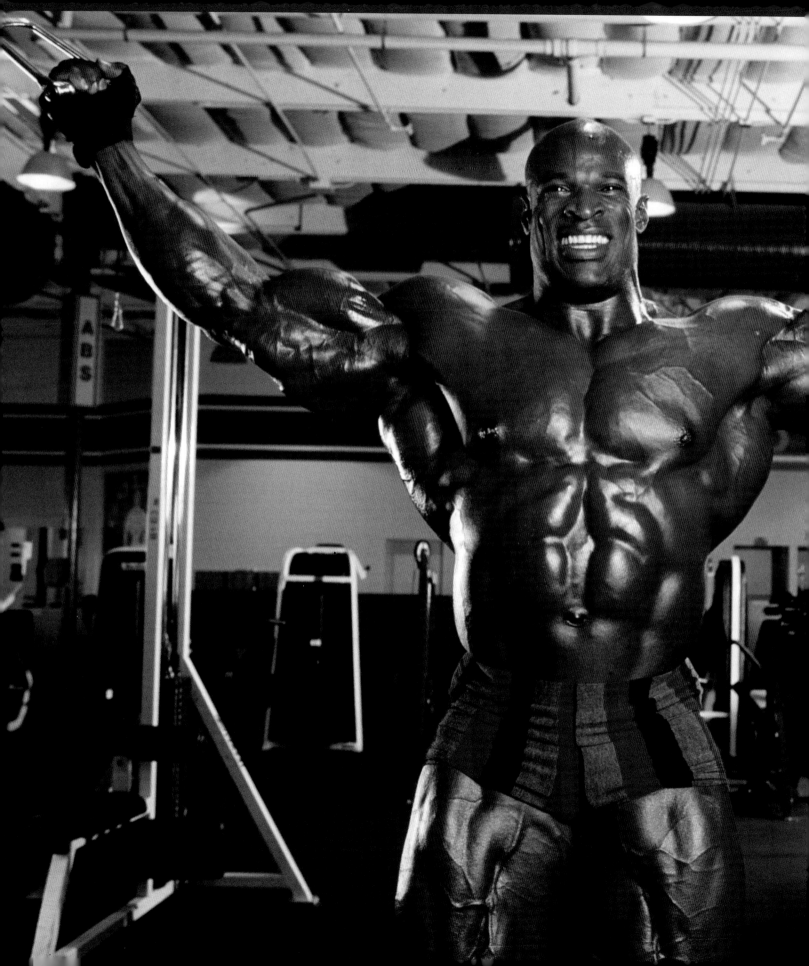

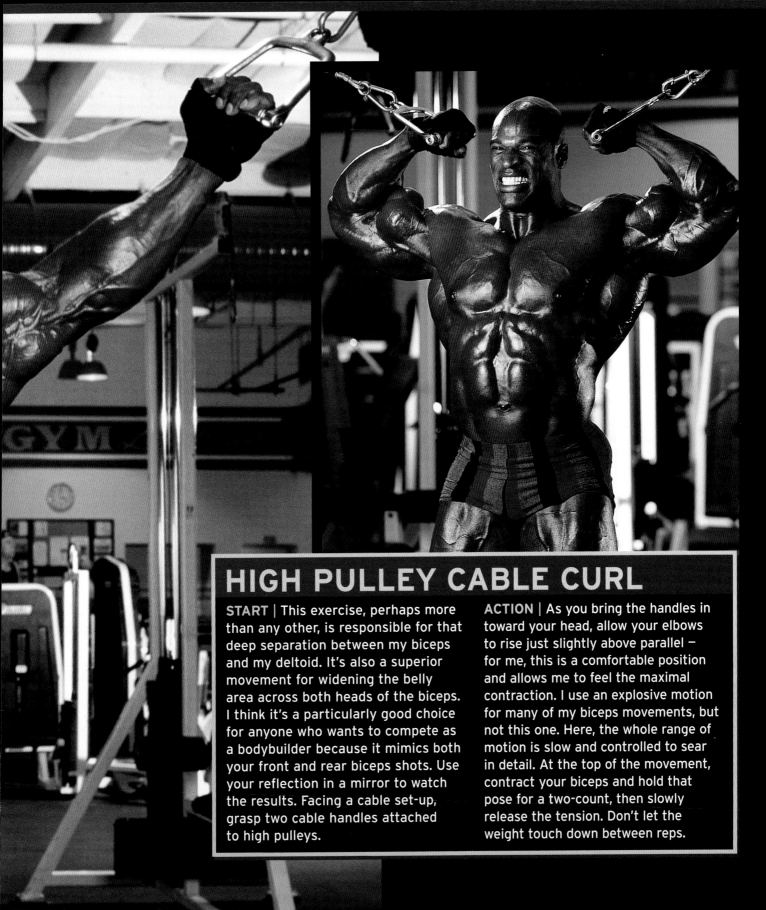

HIGH PULLEY CABLE CURL

START | This exercise, perhaps more than any other, is responsible for that deep separation between my biceps and my deltoid. It's also a superior movement for widening the belly area across both heads of the biceps. I think it's a particularly good choice for anyone who wants to compete as a bodybuilder because it mimics both your front and rear biceps shots. Use your reflection in a mirror to watch the results. Facing a cable set-up, grasp two cable handles attached to high pulleys.

ACTION | As you bring the handles in toward your head, allow your elbows to rise just slightly above parallel – for me, this is a comfortable position and allows me to feel the maximal contraction. I use an explosive motion for many of my biceps movements, but not this one. Here, the whole range of motion is slow and controlled to sear in detail. At the top of the movement, contract your biceps and hold that pose for a two-count, then slowly release the tension. Don't let the weight touch down between reps.

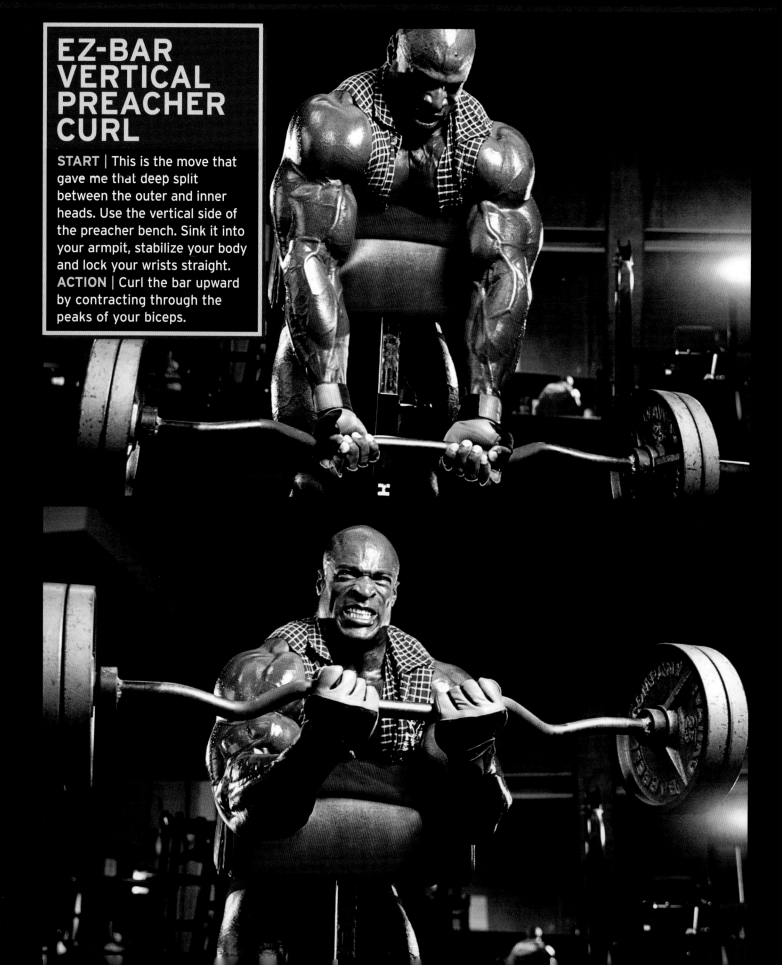

EZ-BAR VERTICAL PREACHER CURL

START | This is the move that gave me that deep split between the outer and inner heads. Use the vertical side of the preacher bench. Sink it into your armpit, stabilize your body and lock your wrists straight.
ACTION | Curl the bar upward by contracting through the peaks of your biceps.

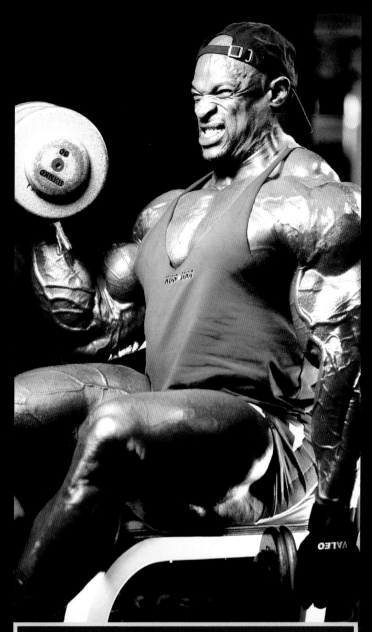

BENT-OVER ONE-ARM CABLE CONCENTRATION CURL

START | For hitting one biceps at a time, and for keeping tension on the muscle all the way through the range of motion, it's hard to beat cable concentration curls. Grasp a D-handle attached to a low pulley and take a solid, staggered stance in front of the apparatus. If possible, place your other hand against the machine or another sturdy object for support.
ACTION | Curl the handle up toward your shoulder, squeeze the muscle as hard as you can, then extend your arm. Complete all reps for one side before switching hands and going through the same drill with the other.

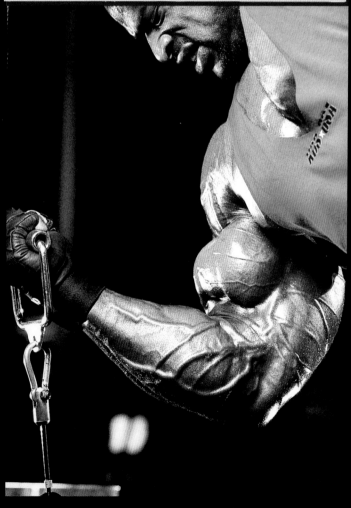

SEATED ALTERNATE DUMBBELL CURL

START | Sit with a dumbbell in each hand, palms facing you, upper arms pressed against your side so your elbow is the only joint working.
ACTION | Feel the outside of your biceps cramp and pump as you twist your wrist while you curl all the way to a peak contraction. (Your palms should face the ceiling at the top.) Squeeze and hold for a second. Resist hard as you slowly lower the dumbbell to a full extension at the bottom. Alternate repetitions, one arm, then the other, until you complete the set.

Ronnie's Biceps Lessons

1 I'VE ALWAYS HAD GREAT BICEPS. When I was young, they were my best bodypart. I trained them all the time, and they seemed as big as my head. I looked kind of funny because they threw off my symmetry, so I finally reduced my training volume from twice a week to once a week to once every other week and finally down to once a month while I allowed the rest of my body to catch up.

2 EVEN THOUGH I HAVE a lot of detail in my biceps, I think about my biceps complex as just one muscle, rather than trying to hit one of the two heads distinctly. When I train biceps, I concentrate on overall movement rather than the movement of individual parts of the muscle structure. When I train my biceps – or any body-part – I think about performance. That's always first and foremost on my mind. I think about getting a good stretch at the bottom of the movement and a strong con-traction at the top. That's what bodybuilding is all about.

3 HAVING SAID THAT, you do need to give some attention to the brachialis muscle, which lies directly beneath the biceps brachii and helps give your upper arm overall volume when developed. The way you hit the brachialis is with hammer-grip movements, palms facing each other. That can be dumbbell hammer curls (standing or seated), rope cable curls or even barbell curls with the specially designed barbell that allows for a hammer-style grip.

4 I START BICEPS TRAINING with a couple of warm-up sets and slowly pyramid up in weight. I typically do three working sets per exercise for arms, with 10 reps minimum each, preferably 12–15, but still pyramiding up in weight even though I'm not backing off on reps. With my peak weight, I strive to hit failure by the time I reach 12 reps or so.

5 DURING ALTERNATING EXERCISES, such as alternating dumbbell curls, don't let the tension totally release on the non-working arm. When one arm is at your side and the other is working, keep that arm at your side tensed. During a set for biceps or for any other muscle group, your body should be fully engaged, all muscles firing – if they're not working, they should be busy stabilizing. That way, you keep your intensity high and your body primed for work. Allowing certain parts of your body to rest lowers your overall energy output and leads to a less productive workout.

6 DON'T BOUNCE OUT OF the bottom of a rep, or lose control of the negative portion of any repetition. As I'll mention again in the upcoming triceps chapter, letting your elbows go to full extension and beyond against resistance can lead to elbow pain and injury over the long haul. If you can't control the weight on the descent and stop just short of lockout, you're probably trying to go too heavy; back off the weight a little and focus on learning proper form.

7 WHILE I DIDN'T INCLUDE chin-ups or Hammer-Strength close-grip pulldowns in the list of alternate exercises for this chapter, they're great biceps exercises, especially if you're desperately trying to build more mass. Chins provide an excellent way to put your bi's under maximum tension and allow you to use your own bodyweight as resistance. Grab the pull-up bar with an underhand grip, just about shoulder-width apart, and concentrate on your biceps when you pull – feel and see them contract as your elbows bend.

8 EXPERIMENT WITH DIFFERENT hand positions and grips. If you look at the exercises I've shown in this chapter, as well as the entire gamut of biceps exercises that exist, you'll see they all have one thing in common: They boil down to your elbows bending against resistance. But for simple variety, and to emphasize different areas of your biceps, exercise variations come in handy. Also, by just changing your grip on a particular exercise, you can add a new twist to your training and perceptibly change which muscle fibers are being hit hardest. On the seated dumbbell curl, for instance, you can go the traditional route, curling from a palms-facing-you position to palms-up at the top; or keep your palms up through-out; or keep your palms hammer-style throughout; or even try a palms-down curl, which engages the biceps and forearms. In any biceps exercise, as long as a curl is at the heart of it, you're doing the job.

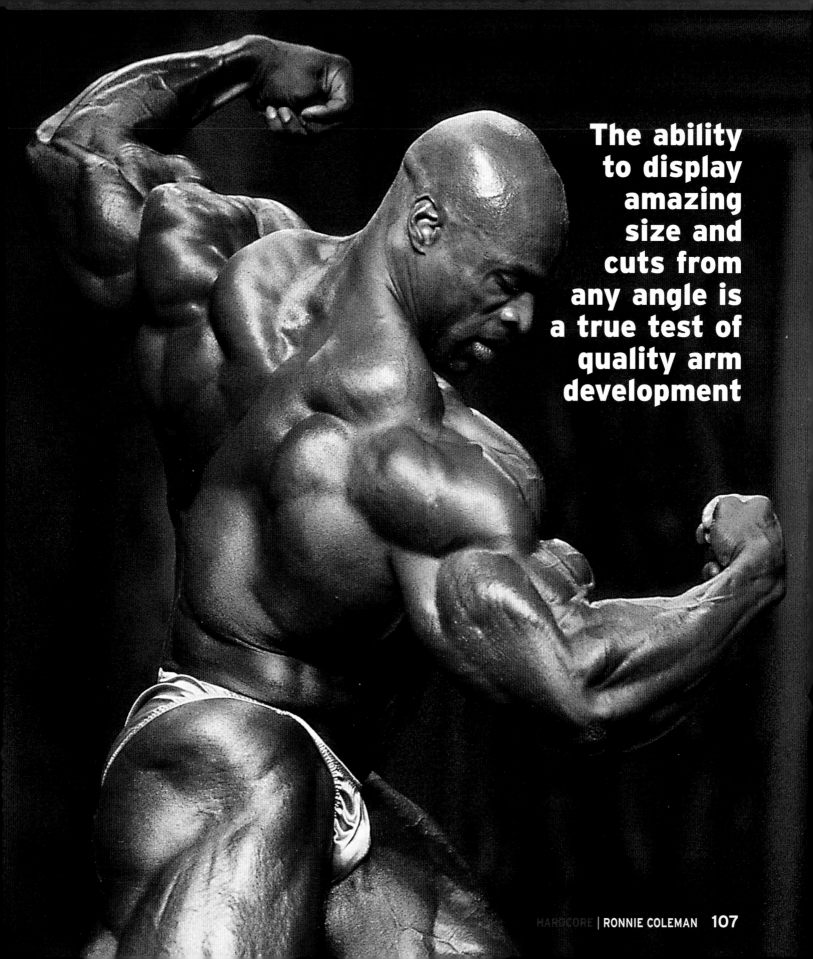

The ability to display amazing size and cuts from any angle is a true test of quality arm development

CHAPTER 7

TITANIC TRICEPS

Triceps are more than just "that other muscle" in your arms. For those of you who shortchange tri's in favor of your biceps, you're not only doing a big disservice to your guns but to your chest and shoulders as well.

I've created my upper-body mass on basics like flat-bench and military presses, going heavy and hard, week after week, month after month, year after muscle-building year. Over time I've been able to peak at about 500 pounds for as many as eight reps on bench presses. But I'd be at a loss to handle the heavy plates on those chest and delt exercises without having first built a solid pair of triceps.

So, with that in mind, you should understand why you need to give your tri's ample attention. Here is the attack I use — put it to work for you and you'll soon be increasing the weight totals in your upper-body lifts, while building impressive arms in the process.

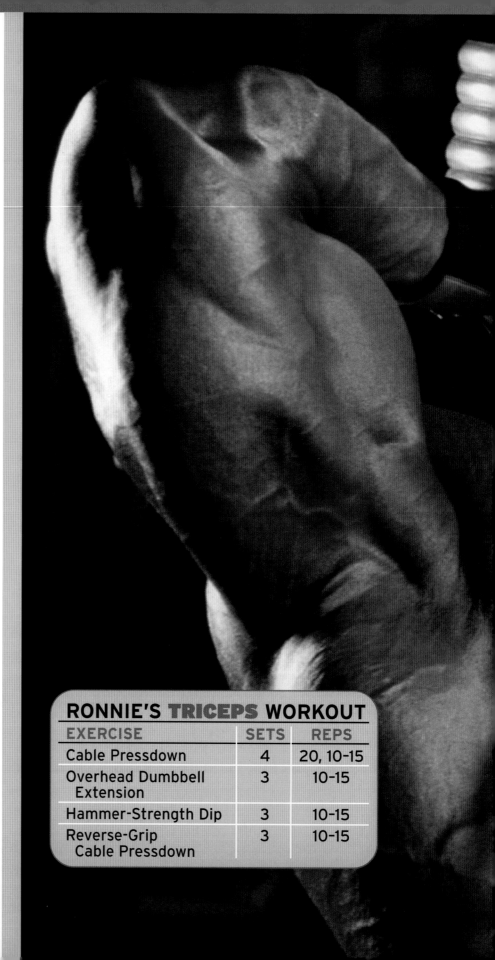

WHILE I WILL VARY MY EXERCISE SELECTION on triceps (check out the "Alternates" section in this chapter for ideas), the four moves built into this workout are the key players.

First up, pressdowns. I see many people bringing up the bar too high and moving their feet all over the place because they're going too heavy without proper stability in their stance. I use a shoulder-width stance, often putting one foot in front of the other for added support if I'm going really heavy. Because this is the first triceps exercise of the day, I perform a light warm-up set of 20 reps, then go into sets of 10–15 reps the rest of the way, always pyramiding up the weight set-to-set on each triceps exercise in the program.

When I do overhead dumbbell extensions, I like to go heavy. I usually start with 130 pounders and go up to 160 or higher over three working sets, trying not to fall below 12 reps at any point. This is one of my favorite exercises because it places maximum tension on the triceps at the point of contraction — where the dumbbells are lowered directly behind your head.

As an alternative, you can also try these one arm at a time. This unilateral blaster can be a key player in helping you overcome strength imbalances; such balance is essential,preparing both of your triceps for the heavy pec-and-delt pushing movements that will make or break your physique.

The third move presented in this workout, the Hammer-Strength dip machine, is awesome for power-building. I suggest you take advantage if you have one of these in your gym, but if not, you can substitute with weighted dips. In this particular workout, I finish with reverse-grip cable pressdowns. I put these last because you have to go lighter, and they're much more of a shaping movement than a mass maker.

RONNIE'S TRICEPS WORKOUT

EXERCISE	SETS	REPS
Cable Pressdown	4	20, 10-15
Overhead Dumbbell Extension	3	10-15
Hammer-Strength Dip	3	10-15
Reverse-Grip Cable Pressdown	3	10-15

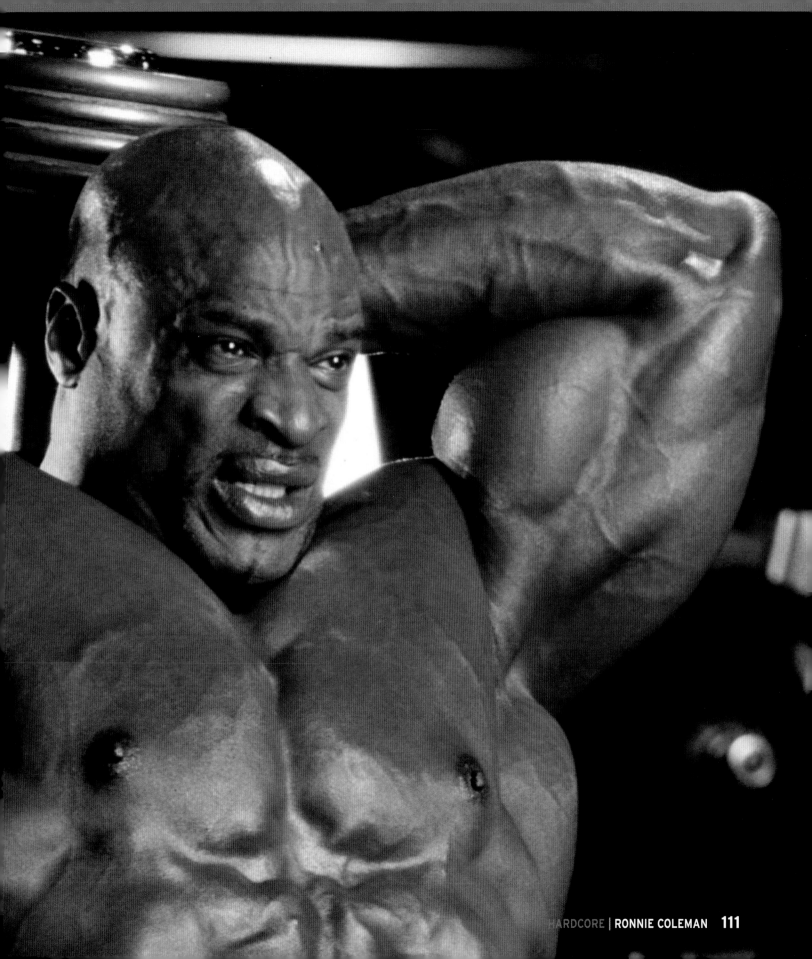

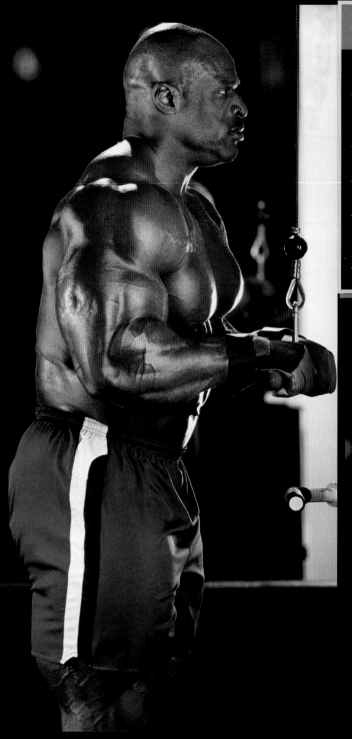

CABLE PRESSDOWN

START | Stand facing a cable machine and take an overhand grip on a straight-bar attachment hooked to the upper pulley. (I'll almost always use a straight bar. The V-shaped handles and cambered bars don't give me the same feeling of power and as complete a contraction as the straight bar does.) Start with the bar at about lower chest level and press your elbows in close to your sides.

ACTION | From here, forcibly press the bar down toward the floor, contracting hard through your triceps and stopping just short of locking out. Pause a moment and squeeze in this fully contracted position before moving to the negative, resisting the pull of the cable on the return.

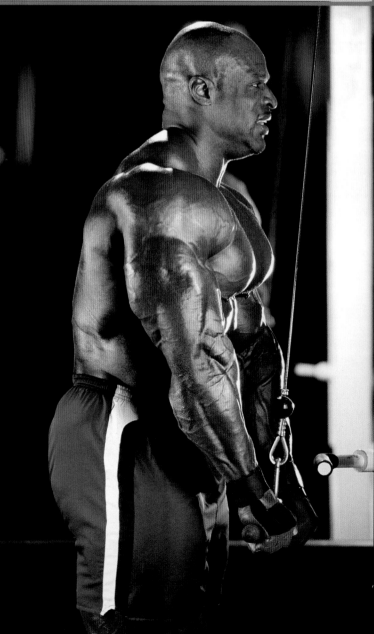

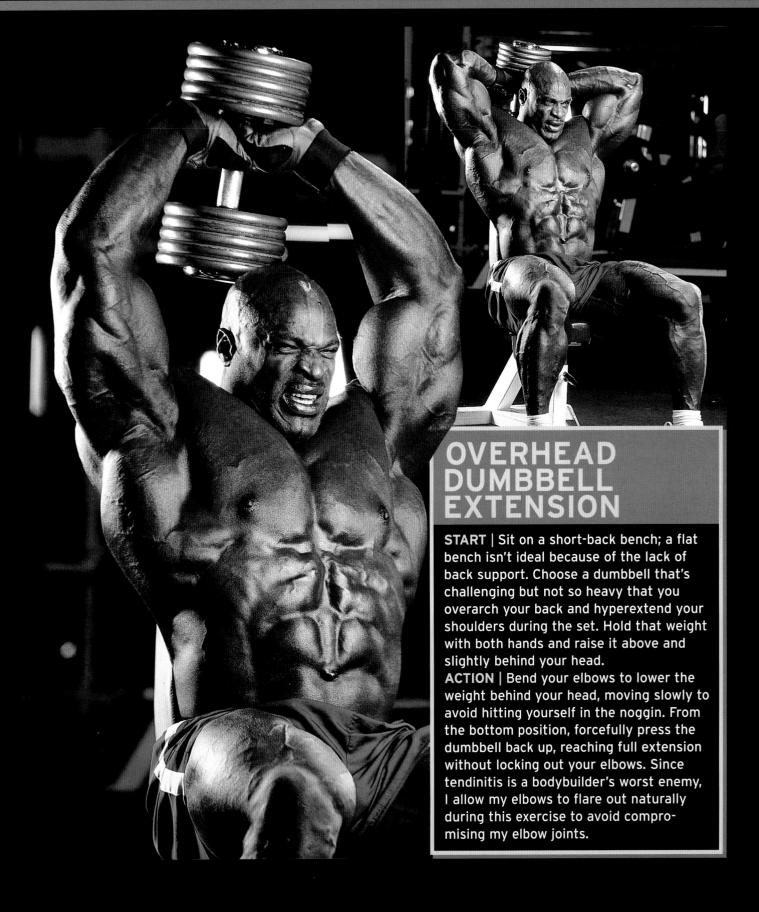

OVERHEAD DUMBBELL EXTENSION

START | Sit on a short-back bench; a flat bench isn't ideal because of the lack of back support. Choose a dumbbell that's challenging but not so heavy that you overarch your back and hyperextend your shoulders during the set. Hold that weight with both hands and raise it above and slightly behind your head.

ACTION | Bend your elbows to lower the weight behind your head, moving slowly to avoid hitting yourself in the noggin. From the bottom position, forcefully press the dumbbell back up, reaching full extension without locking out your elbows. Since tendinitis is a bodybuilder's worst enemy, I allow my elbows to flare out naturally during this exercise to avoid compromising my elbow joints.

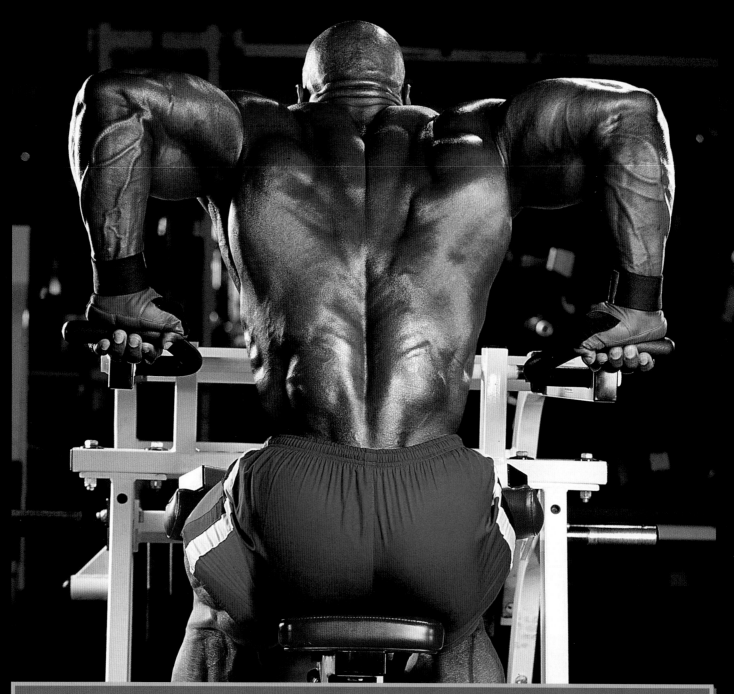

HAMMER-STRENGTH DIP

START | Sit backwards on a dip machine and plant your feet on the floor in front of you. I like to sit backwards on the machine because the angle puts a greater emphasis on my triceps, all but taking the chest out of the equation. Take a firm grip on the machine handles and bring your elbows in close to your body.

ACTION | Press down forcibly on the handles, keeping your elbows in close as you reach full elbow extension without completely locking out. Slowly reverse the motion and resist the push of the handles on the return, stopping just short of the weights coming to rest.

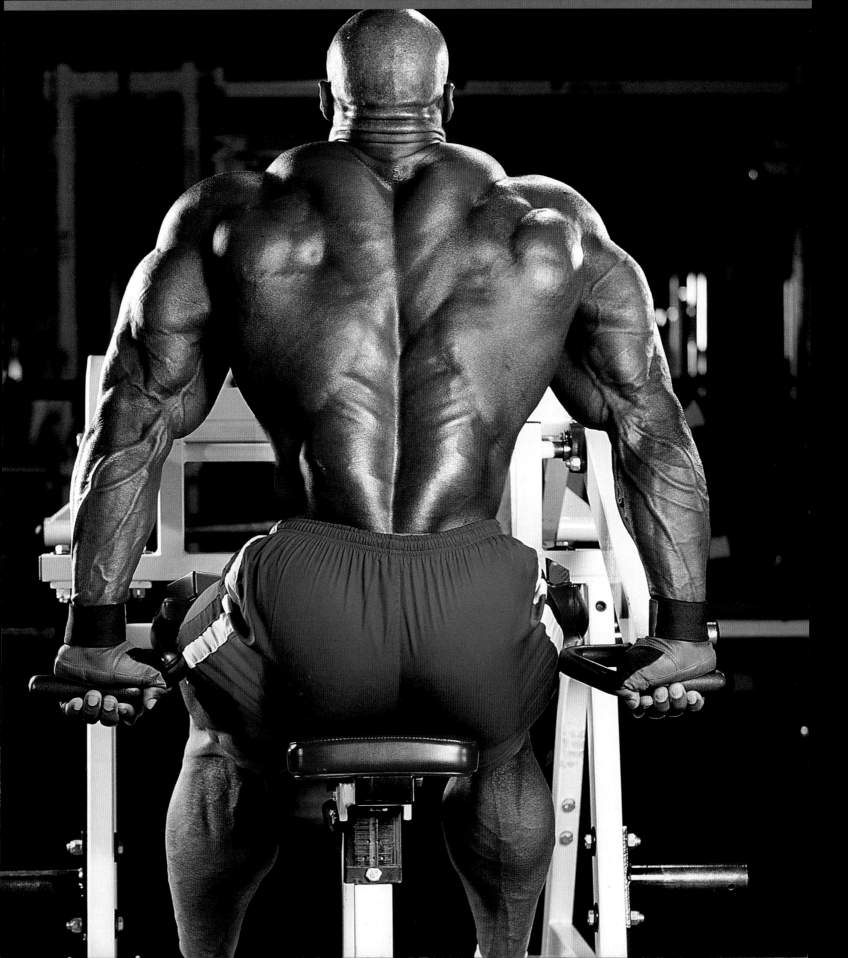

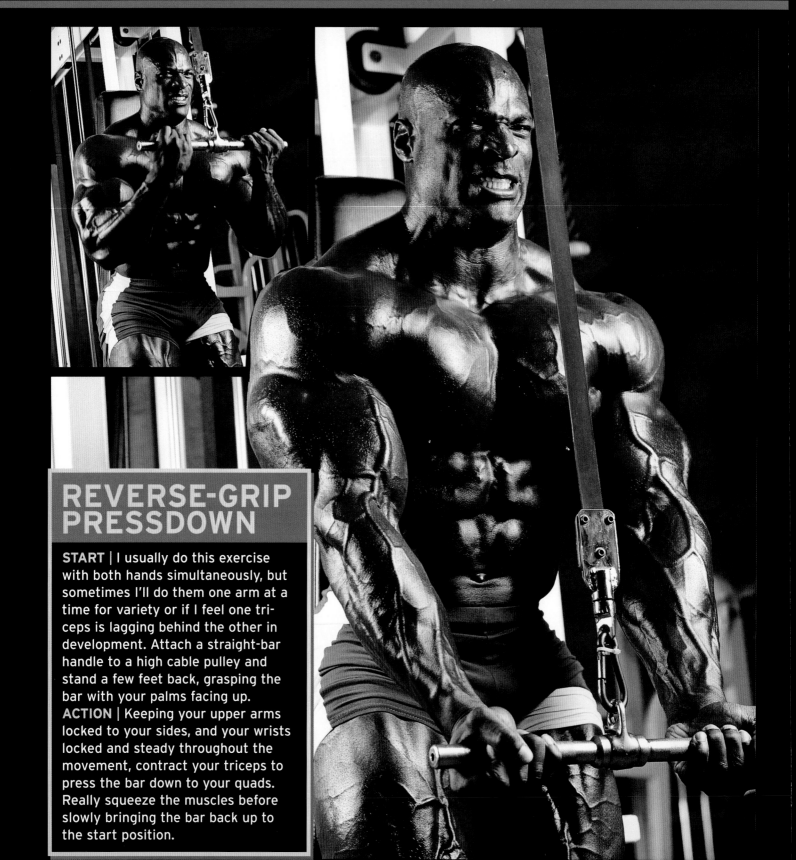

REVERSE-GRIP PRESSDOWN

START | I usually do this exercise with both hands simultaneously, but sometimes I'll do them one arm at a time for variety or if I feel one triceps is lagging behind the other in development. Attach a straight-bar handle to a high cable pulley and stand a few feet back, grasping the bar with your palms facing up.

ACTION | Keeping your upper arms locked to your sides, and your wrists locked and steady throughout the movement, contract your triceps to press the bar down to your quads. Really squeeze the muscles before slowly bringing the bar back up to the start position.

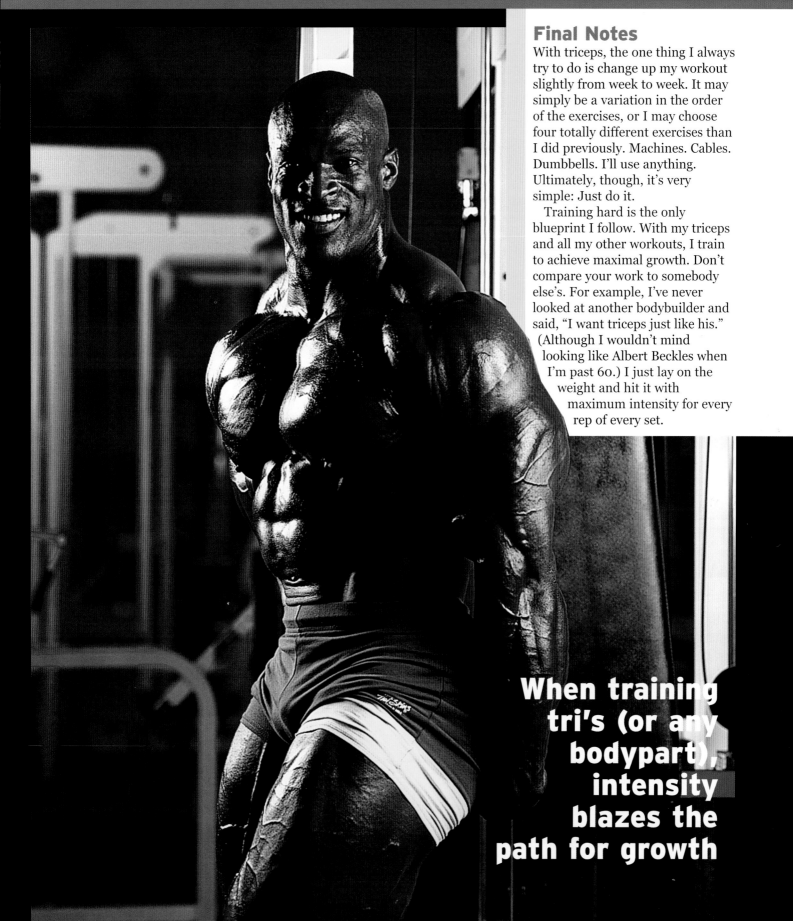

Final Notes

With triceps, the one thing I always try to do is change up my workout slightly from week to week. It may simply be a variation in the order of the exercises, or I may choose four totally different exercises than I did previously. Machines. Cables. Dumbbells. I'll use anything. Ultimately, though, it's very simple: Just do it.

Training hard is the only blueprint I follow. With my triceps and all my other workouts, I train to achieve maximal growth. Don't compare your work to somebody else's. For example, I've never looked at another bodybuilder and said, "I want triceps just like his." (Although I wouldn't mind looking like Albert Beckles when I'm past 60.) I just lay on the weight and hit it with maximum intensity for every rep of every set.

When training tri's (or any bodypart), intensity blazes the path for growth

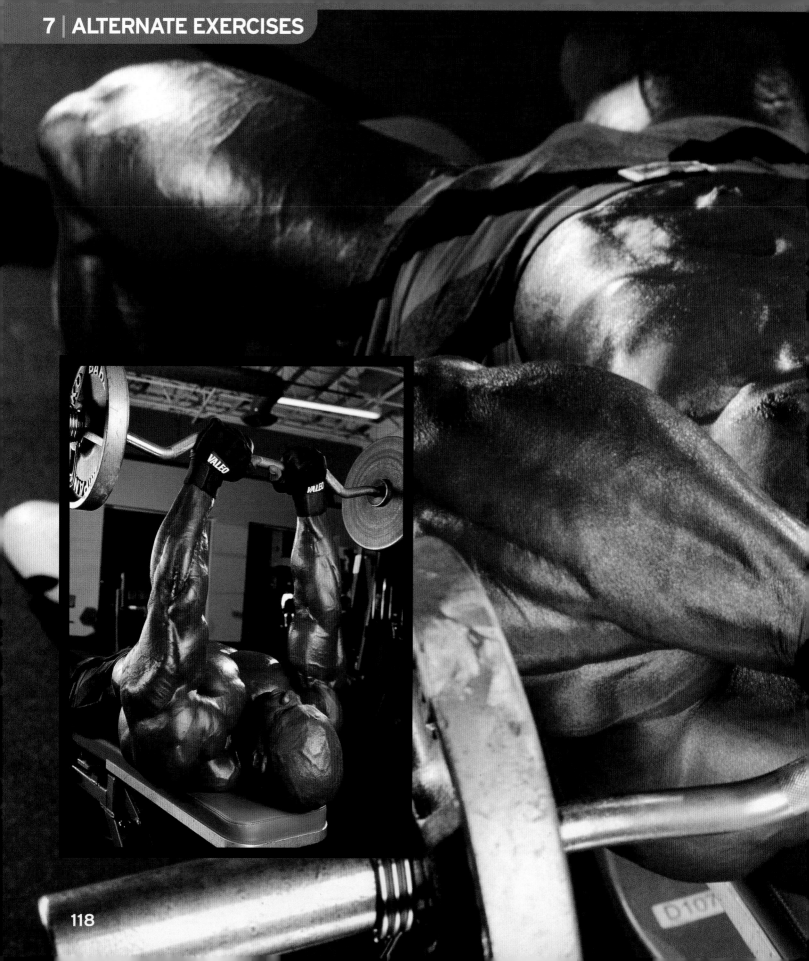

LYING FRENCH PRESS

START | Lie on a bench with your feet flat on the floor, your lower back pressed firmly into the padding. Grasp an EZ-bar with an overhand grip. Begin the movement with your arms extended straight above your body.

ACTION | Slowly lower the weight by bending at your elbow joint, keeping your upper arms and the rest of your body steady as the bar travels toward your forehead. Then reverse direction by contracting your tri's to power the bar back upward.

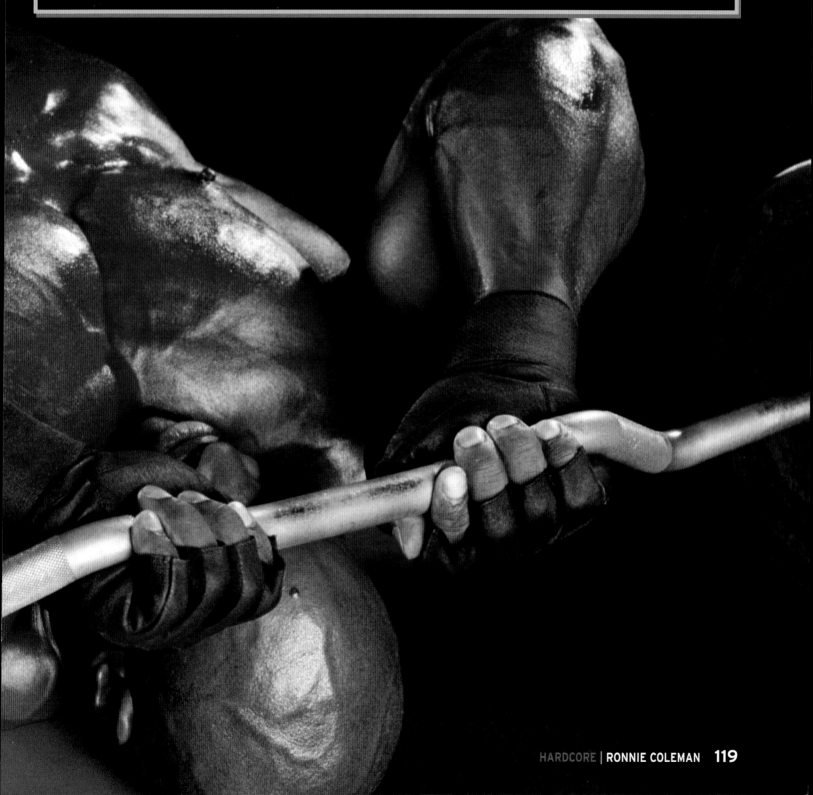

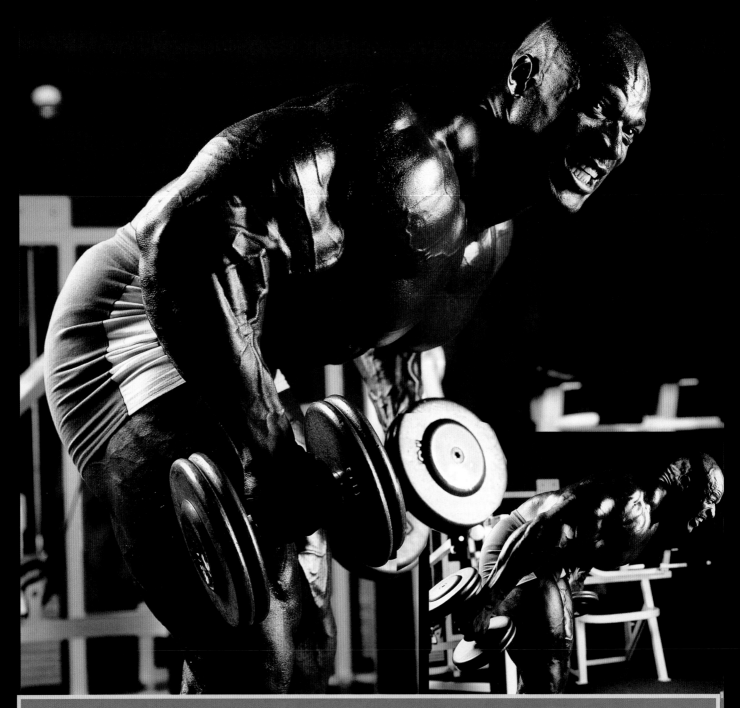

DUMBBELL KICKBACK

START | I know a lot of people do these one side at a time, but I like training both arms simultaneously to ensure that I don't twist or tweak my torso like I tend to do when I single them out. Grasp a pair of dumbbells and lean forward with your knees slightly bent, back flat and abs tight. Pin your upper arms to your sides, keeping them there throughout the move.

ACTION | Allowing the weights to hang straight down at the beginning, elbows fully bent, lift both dumbbells back and up while turning your palms outward and upward just a little bit. The muscles are fully contracted when your arms are straight; briefly hold that peak contraction before slowly lowering the weights to the start.

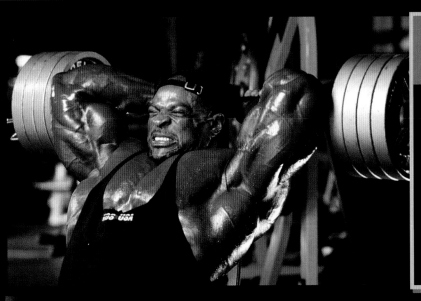

SEATED EZ-BAR EXTENSION

START | Sit on a low-back bench and have a spotter hand you the weight, balancing it for you as you take a grasp on the bar on the inner curl.

ACTION | From that point, drive the bar hard to lift it straight up overhead, stopping just before your elbows lock out and then returning to the bottom. This exercise puts your triceps on an extreme stretch, so take it slowly and don't load up with a heavy weight right off the bat.

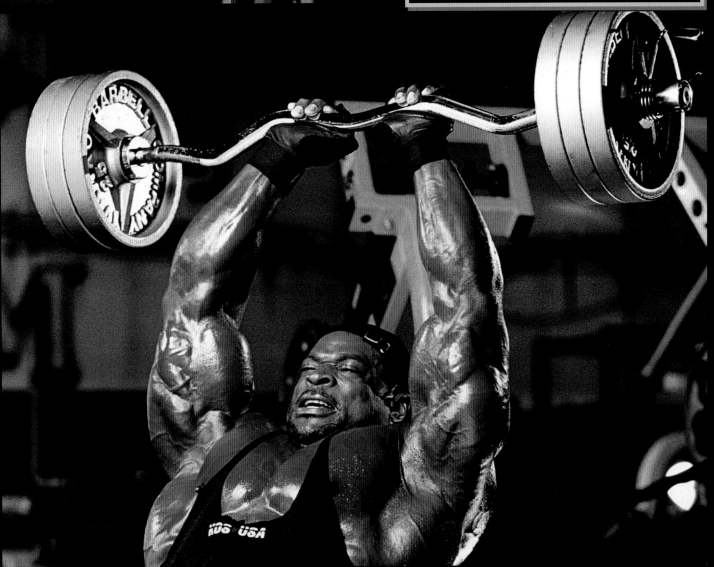

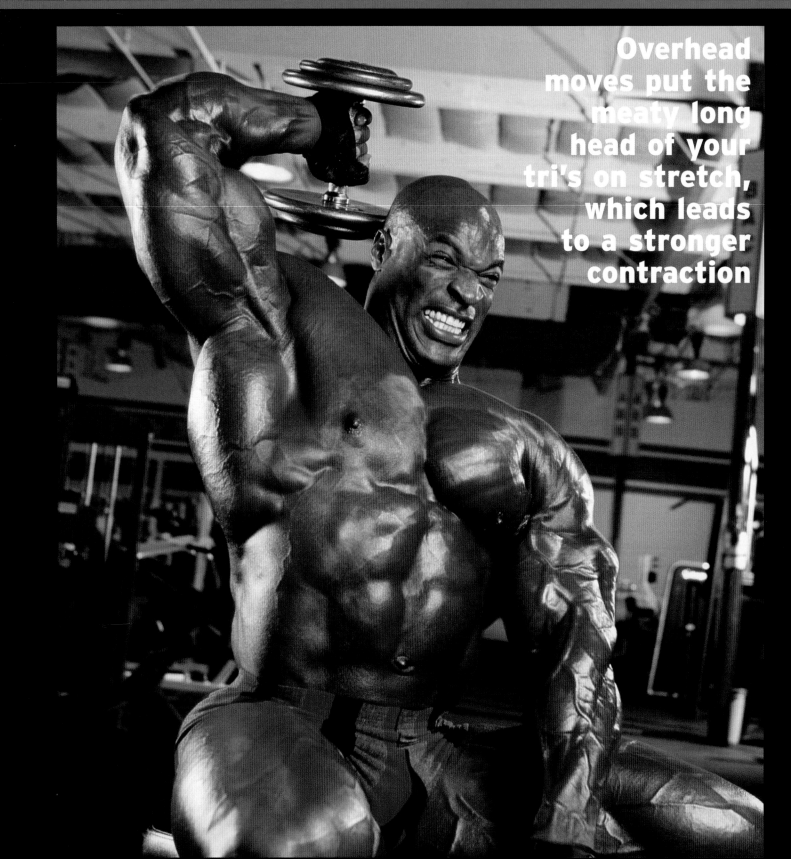

Overhead moves put the meaty long head of your tri's on stretch, which leads to a stronger contraction

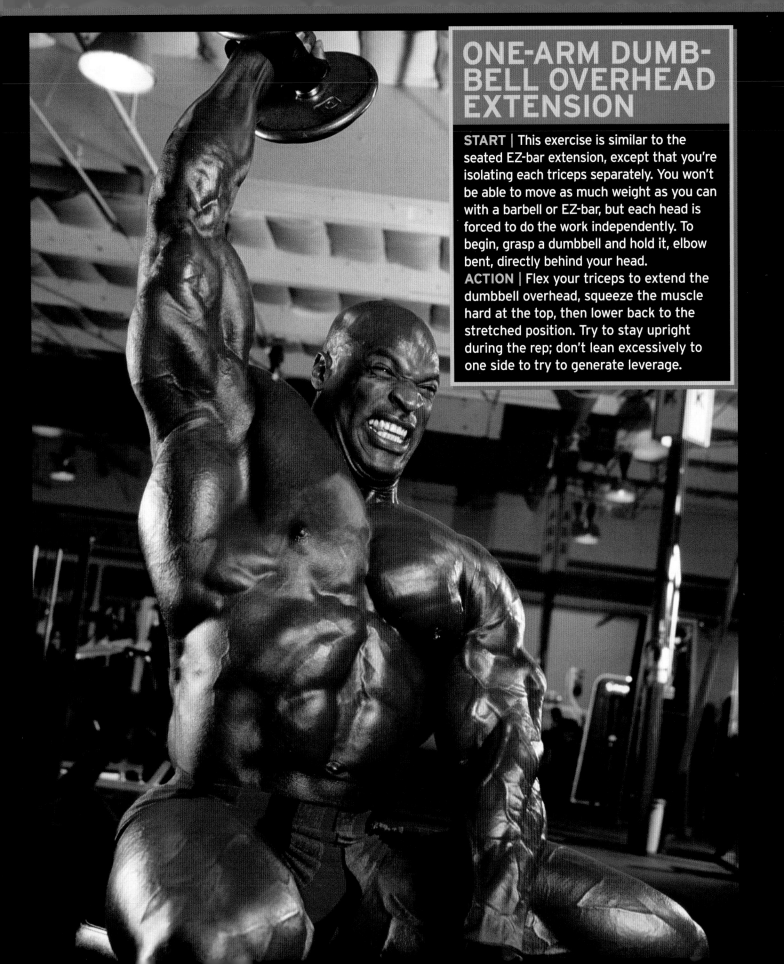

ONE-ARM DUMB-BELL OVERHEAD EXTENSION

START | This exercise is similar to the seated EZ-bar extension, except that you're isolating each triceps separately. You won't be able to move as much weight as you can with a barbell or EZ-bar, but each head is forced to do the work independently. To begin, grasp a dumbbell and hold it, elbow bent, directly behind your head.

ACTION | Flex your triceps to extend the dumbbell overhead, squeeze the muscle hard at the top, then lower back to the stretched position. Try to stay upright during the rep; don't lean excessively to one side to try to generate leverage.

CLOSE-GRIP BENCH PRESS

START | The close-grip press is a solid way to start off a triceps workout. It's just like a bench press, except you take a grip on the bar where your hands are 8–12 inches apart.

ACTION | Lower the bar to your chest, then press it back up. Bring your elbows in closer to better recruit your triceps, and space your hands far enough apart that you don't feel pain in your wrists.

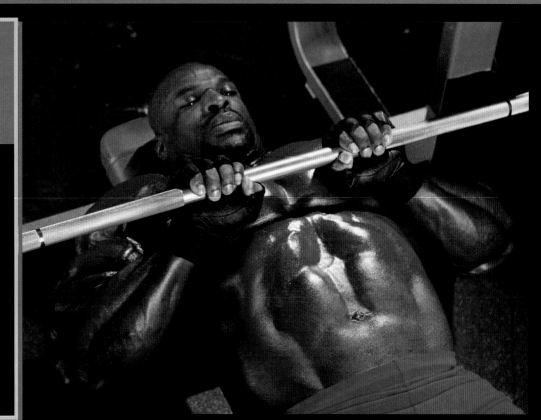

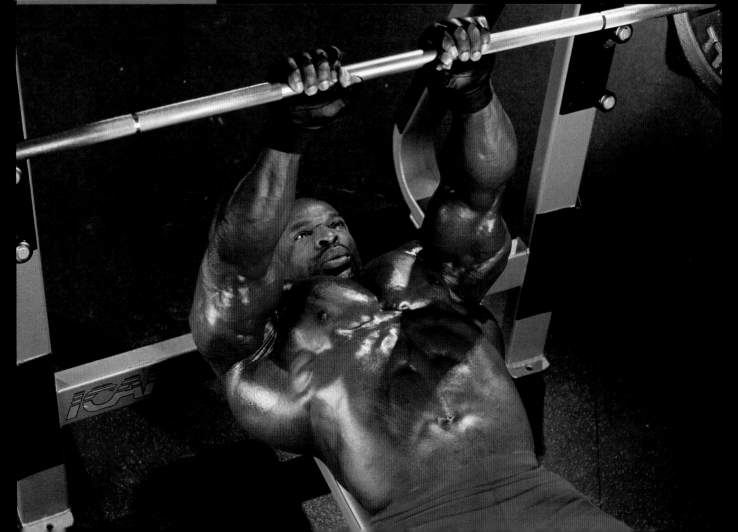

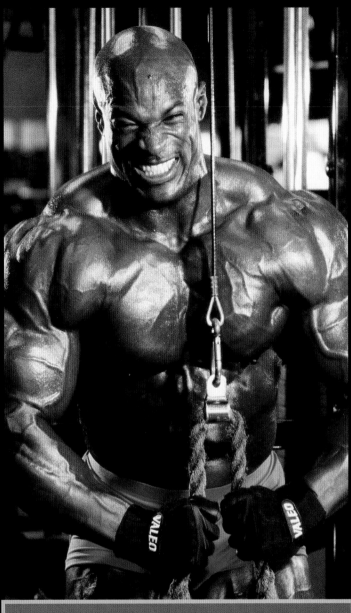

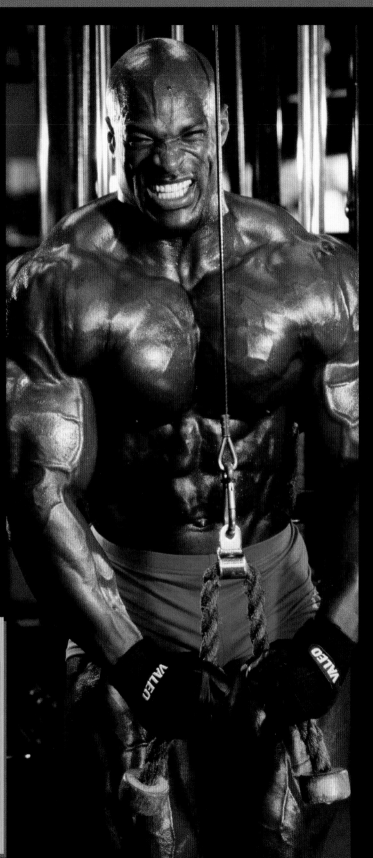

ROPE PRESSDOWN

START | This move is just like a cable pressdown with a straight bar, except you're using a rope, which provides more of a hammer-style grip and slightly changes the feel of the exercise in your triceps. To begin, grasp a rope firmly. Here, you can see I took hold of the rope away from the ends, but you can also grasp the ends so your pinkies are right up against the knots or stoppers.

ACTION | Moving only at your elbow joint, press the rope down, then return under control to the start.

Ronnie's Triceps Lessons

1 WHEN TRAINING ARMS, I use different exercises every week to keep things fresh and to continue making progress. For example, instead of doing overhead dumbbell extensions, I'll do lying french presses or the seated EZ-bar extension. Also, I don't have a set order in which I do my triceps exercises, nor do I have a plan I follow on any given day. I'll pick an exercise that feels natural to start with and jump on in. But no matter what, I'll always do at least one warm-up set with that initial motion to pump some blood into the muscle and get it ready to work.

2 I NEVER LOCK OUT ANY JOINT, especially not my elbows. The elbows are very vulnerable joints, and forcing them to lock out compromises all the ligaments and tendons that cross that area. To ensure that I get a full, complete contraction, I use mental power. Yes, you want to make sure you hit a peak contraction with each triceps movement, but the key is trying to do it without completely locking out your elbow. In other words, find the "sweet spot" where your triceps are fully engaged, yet you haven't completely put your elbow on lockdown, or worse yet, slightly hyperextended it. Pause, and squeeze the muscle momentarily before releasing. Learning this nuance of triceps training is half your battle in the quest for bigger guns.

3 EVERYONE WANTS BIG PIPES, but almost no one goes about it correctly. You'll see guys in the gym training arms every day, trying to make them bigger, but what they're really doing is over-training and causing them to shrink. If you want growth in your arms, train your biceps and triceps no more than twice a week, using proper and complete contractions, and go as heavy as possible without compromising your form. It's that simple.

4 THE TRICEPS IS THE LARGER of the two arm muscle groups, and I feel that means it can handle more training than the biceps. However, if you spend 45 minutes training triceps, you're probably over-training them. If your arms aren't responding well, look to add intensity, not more sets, to your workout. (See tips Nos. 7 and 8 for some intensity-boosting ideas.)

5 HIT ALL THREE TRICEPS HEADS in your workout, but know which exercises stress particular areas the greatest. For instance, the long head is targeted with moves that put your triceps on stretch, such as during overhead dumbbell extensions and the lying french press. The medial and lateral heads are emphasized when your arms are at your sides, such as with the many variations of cable pressdowns. Spend some time learning new exercises and include movements that work your arms in different ways in each workout.

6 I HAD GOOD TRICEPS FROM THE BEGINNING, and I was lucky enough to have some people take me under their wings who knew what they were doing. I also had a head start because of my powerlifting background. But you don't need the same type of head start to see fast results. When I began bodybuilding, I relied on multiple sets, a 10-15 rep range, and limited rest periods of 30-90 seconds between sets; it was a simple philosophy that paid dividends.

7 TO SQUEEZE A LITTLE MORE out of your workout, try some intensity-raising techniques. For instance, you could try to compound-set the exercises in your workout; in the routine presented in this chapter, you could pair Hammer-Strength dips and overhead dumbbell extensions at the start of your session, then finish off with cable pressdowns and reverse pressdowns. In a compound set, exercises are performed back to back with no rest in between. So you would do 10-15 reps of the Hammer-Strength dip, then immediately grab a dumbbell with both hands and complete 10-15 reps of overhead extensions. Rest a minute, then go into the second compound set, rest another minute, and do one final compound set before moving onto the two cable moves.

8 DROP SETS ARE ANOTHER GOOD intensity technique for triceps. Say you're on the cable pressdown: Choose a heavy weight and go for failure at around 12 reps, then quickly reset the pin 10-20 pounds lighter and keep going until failure. Getting 3-4 drops in your final set will leave no muscle fiber unturned when you're through and ready to head home.

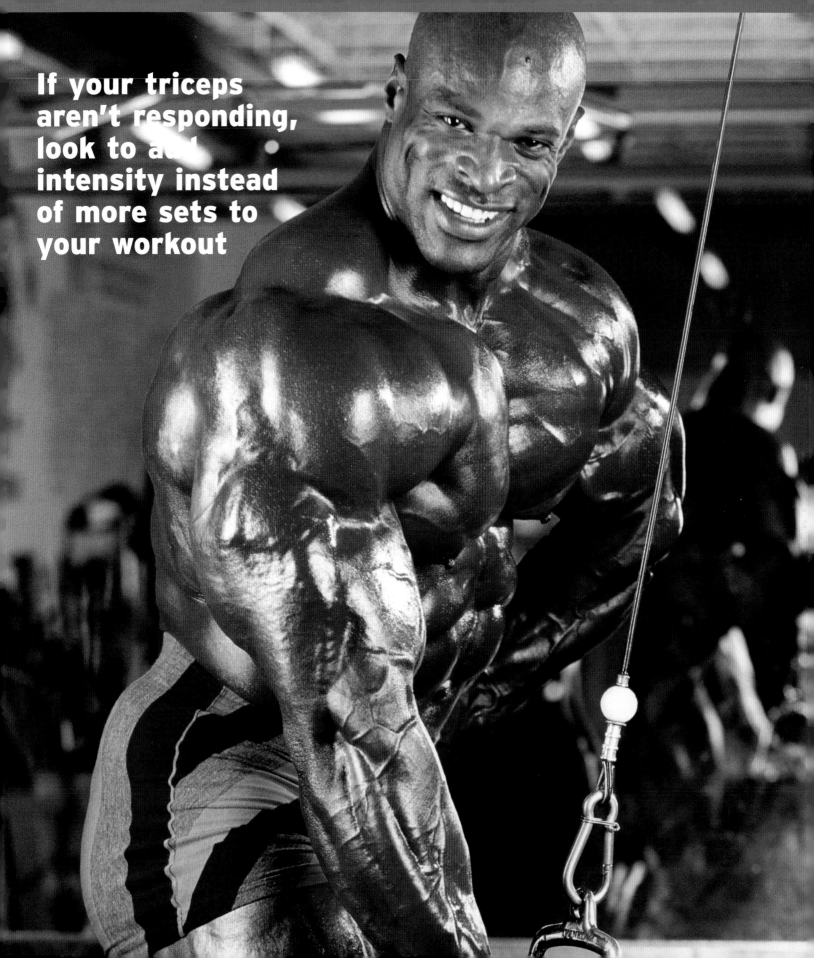

If your triceps aren't responding, look to add intensity instead of more sets to your workout

CHAPTER 8

TRAINING CYCLE

The more I change, the more everything remains the same. In other words, the more I grow, the more convinced I am that what I'm doing is what works best, and the less likely I am to change it.

That's a common-sense approach to anything in life but an especially sure-fire formula for bodybuilding. So for all of my valued fans out there who beg me to reveal a fresh new secret for maximizing off-season growth, here's my advice: Beware of the slick and quick. Instead, dig in, tether yourself to the basics, and forge ahead. It's tried and true, and it's what I do.

With that said, here is a sample of how I might put my training together for a year leading up to a contest. As a rule, my approach doesn't change much leading up to a show. While some other bodybuilders radically change their training philosophy in the 6-12 weeks before a show, I don't. What works for gaining mass should work as well for refining it; the real secret is in the manipulation of your diet, although I don't go overboard there either, as you'll see in Chapter 9.

As I mentioned in the bodypart-focused chapters, while there are bread-and-butter exercises I stick to, I do try to work some variety into my routine. Thus, you'll see this program is a bit different than if you simply took the bodypart workouts I provided and combined them. As I said, this is a sample: Every year, in preparation for the Olympia, everything comes together slightly differently. But this will give you an idea of how to structure your own training, whether you're just trying to build a better body or you intend to go the distance and compete as a bona fide bodybuilder.

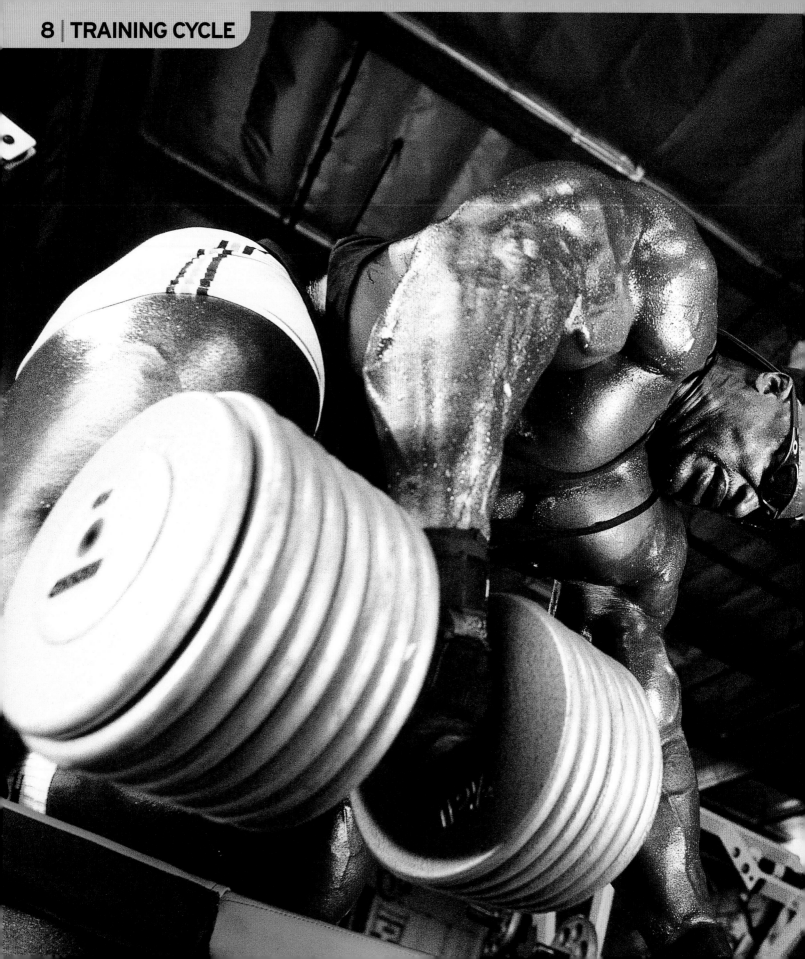

THE PRINCIPLES OF SIZE

Analyze the workouts I'm revealing here, and you'll see that I'm using the same exercises and the same basic principles as I did when I turned pro over a decade ago:

(a) I use extremely heavy poundages;

(b) I employ a higher-rep scheme than what is normally prescribed for bodybuilders;

(c) I hit each bodypart twice a week with alternating workouts, one for power and the other focused on creating muscle separation.

I also want to drive home this point: To me, there's no such thing as precontest training. My off-season routine is my precontest routine. Nothing changes in terms of sets, reps, schedule, you name it, right up to the day of the show. If you've been wondering how I can take the stage with the same amount of mass I carry during the off-season, that explanation should solve the mystery.

Beyond those immutable principles, you'll find that change, itself, is also an important factor, in the sense that no consecutive workouts are exactly the same. Something will change, even if it's as miniscule as repetitions or the angle of an exercise, the reason being that there are more valid training techniques in bodybuilding than can be accommodated in a single workout. So if I throw in a different one every session, I am, over time, utilizing every principle of value without straying from my basic mass-building and refining routine.

My training cycle is six days on, one off, working every bodypart over three days, before starting the cycle again on the fourth day. The first time through (Monday, Tuesday and Wednesday), I train my body with powerlifting movements, compound exercises and very heavy free weights to build mass and power. The second time through (Thursday, Friday and Saturday), I use bodybuilding techniques to develop individual muscles and exaggerate separations. The constant is the reps, which stay in the 10–15 range for all save a few super-heavy sets on powerlifting essentials like deadlifts and squats.

I don't know of any other pro who employs this exact style of training but, without it, a physique will not retain the two essential qualities of muscularity. A strict powerlifting routine will sacrifice separations, and a strict bodybuilding routine will sacrifice mass. By using the former in the first half of the week and the latter in the last half of the week, I integrate the advantages of both extremes into my muscle mass.

MAKING IT COUNT

Regardless of the technique, I count reps for every set, rather than put my faith in failure. The former commits you to a fixed and objective goal; whereas, the latter is determined by your vague whims. A numerical goal won't let either my mind or my body off the hook; but I take it even further. If I set for myself a 10-rep goal, for example, I'll put on enough weight so that it's almost physically impossible for me to complete eight, but I won't stop until I've done at least 12. Somehow, some way, I always find a way to exceed my goal.

To some people, extremely heavy weight with a lot of reps is a paradox, but to me, it's a principle. You need extremely heavy weight to force yourself beyond your boundaries, but you also need repetitions to fully stimulate a muscle in all its fibers.

As for what constitutes too many repetitions, that depends on what it takes to work the intended muscle. If you're getting a surface burn without a deep pump, you're doing too many reps. With leg extensions, for example, I can't get the right pump until I've done at least 30 reps; whereas, when I squat I get my best pump with 10–12 reps.

Whether I'm doing a powerlifting exercise or a bodybuilding exercise, I want to give the muscle a valiant challenge. The burn doesn't have to fry the flesh off my bones, but at least there has to be a hard pull at the muscle insertions and an assurance that the belly of the muscle is being swollen with blood under high pressure. That sensation can't be fully generated unless you use a complete range of motion. Partial reps shouldn't be a major portion of your program. Only a complete extension and a hard peak contraction can hammer that muscle into place.

I'd love to have you follow my training program to the letter, but I'm afraid that's too much to ask. I've found that my recuperative powers are so extraordinary that, about an hour after a workout, I'm again ready to go. Consequently, I have yet to find anyone who can stay with me.

Let's assume, though, that you're the exception. If so, tag along, and if you're still with me at the end of the week, I'll probably see you on the Mr. Olympia stage some day.

My training varies, but there are no "light" days

THE RUNDOWN

Below are some highlights of each of the routines outlined on the following pages.

BACK

You can probably tell by looking at me that I love to work back. I also love deadlifts — so much so that I sometimes go up to 800 pounds with them. That's the reason I schedule my back workout to follow a rest day. I like to dominate my deadlifts, rather than approach them with awe and respect. At the same time, I'm constantly trying to build muscle, so I pyramid up to that max through a lot of 10- to 12-rep sets, starting with one plate on each side of the bar, then adding a plate per set, until I can only get six reps for my penultimate set. After that, I may try to double with 800 pounds.

BICEPS

I use very distinct workouts for biceps: Workout A will most likely be straight sets with free weights; whereas, for workout B, I may go through all of the exercises nonstop, using giant sets, supersets or drop sets. Whichever mode I choose on that "B" day, it'll be extremely intense.

DELTS

The shoulder complex needs to be hit with more heavy techniques than a once-a-week workout can provide, so every workout is an unpredictable mixture of movements. What *is* predictable, however, is that each time I'll use basic, free-weight straight sets but also from time to time giant sets, supersets or drop sets.

The only traditional shoulder exercise I no longer do is behind- the-neck presses. The only reason it became popular in the first place is because it's a position that permits a very powerful piston effect for pressing. Unfortunately, it also imposes destructive stresses on the shoulder complex, which is how I hurt my shoulder a long time ago. Now, I do seated military presses to the front instead, which builds plenty of mass in the deltoids without the same risks.

LEGS

The most unorthodox exercise I do is the parking lot lunges, which I first introduced in the legs chapter. I go outside to the gym parking lot and, with a 135-pound barbell on my back, I'll lunge for about 100 yards to the other end. I then increase the weight to 185 or 225 pounds and lunge back to the starting point.

CHEST

Workouts A and B comprise totally different exercises, yet all are done with barbells and dumbbells. The chest is such a vast muscle group that in order to reach its deepest and most remote fibers, it must be hit with as many compound movements as possible, from every direction, and with the most extreme poundages you can handle through the most extreme ranges of motion. Free weights are the only means of satisfying those criterion, and I use every one of the basics, as you'll see in my workout chart. Here, too, I've discovered that 10-15-rep sets produce the most off-season mass in the shortest time.

TRICEPS

Each triceps workout I do is meant to maximize my mass and hardness. I use a killer combination of basic free-weight and select machine exercises, while employing a number of special techniques to pound the message of growth home: supersets, tri-sets, giant sets, drop sets and double-drop sets are a few of my favorites. In addition, I change the order of exercises often. For me, high reps between 12 and 15 build the most mass in my triceps in the shortest amount of time. If you try my program for yourself, I think you'll like how your body responds.

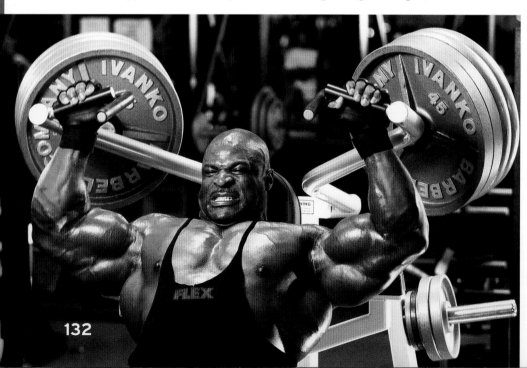

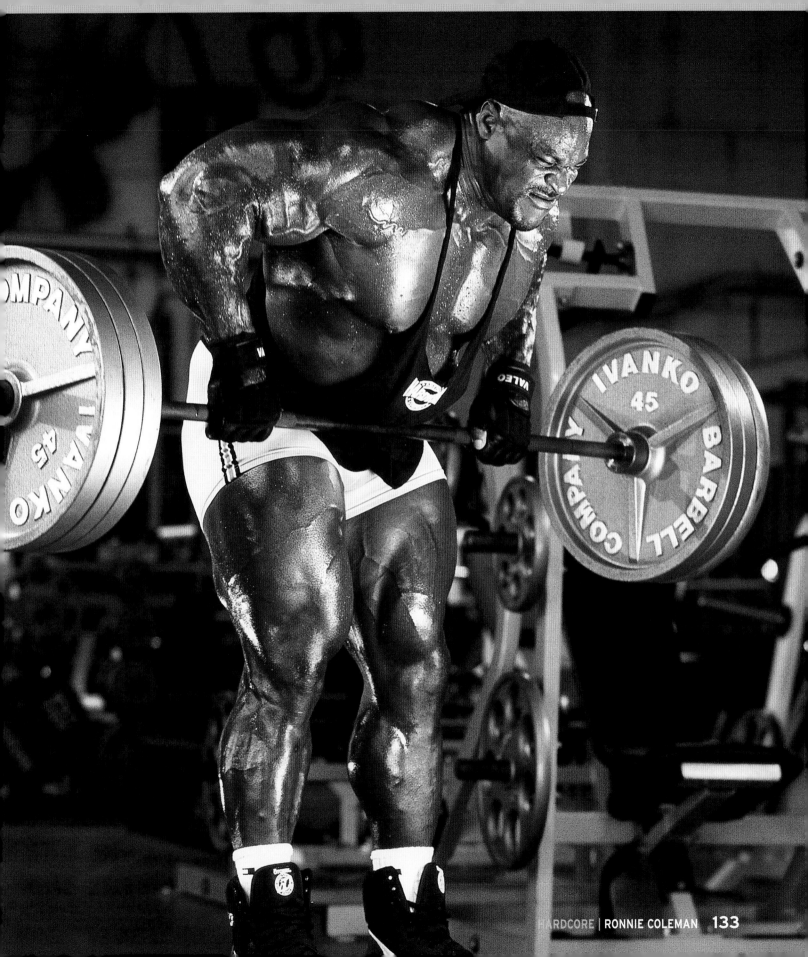

MY OFF-SEASON/PRECONTEST WORKOUT

If you're well past the beginner stage, you can follow my routine or a modified version of it. If you don't want to follow the whole routine, choose two or three exercises for each bodypart and go from there. Follow the routine for six weeks, take a weeklong break, and then commence another six-week cycle. The exercise and sets are listed; reps are in the 10-15 range for every exercise unless listed otherwise.

DAY 1 - MONDAY
Workout A: Back, Biceps, Delts

BACK	
EXERCISE	SETS
Deadlift	4 (15-6 reps)
Bent-Over Barbell Row	4
T-Bar Row	4
One-Arm Dumbbell Row	4
BICEPS	
Standing Barbell Curl	4
Seated Alternate Dumbbell Curl	3
EZ-Bar Preacher Curl	3
Standing Cable Curl	3
DELTS	
Seated Barbell Press	4
Incline Lateral Raise (superset with)	4
Front Dumbbell Raise	4

DAY 2 - TUESDAY
Workout A: Legs

THIGHS	
EXERCISE	SETS
Leg Extension	15–30
Barbell Squat	5
Hack Squat	3
(or) Leg Press	3
Lying Leg Curl	3
Walking Lunge	3
CALVES	
Donkey Calf Raise	4

DAY 3 - WEDNESDAY
Workout A: Chest, Triceps

CHEST	
EXERCISE	SETS
Flat-Bench Barbell Press	4
Incline Barbell Press	3
Decline Barbell Press	3
Pec-Deck Flye	3
TRICEPS	
Cable Pressdown	4
Seated Overhead Dumbbell Extension	3
Hammer-Strength Dip	3
Reverse-Grip Cable Pressdown	3

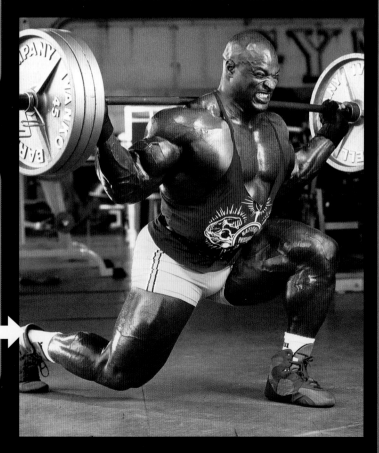

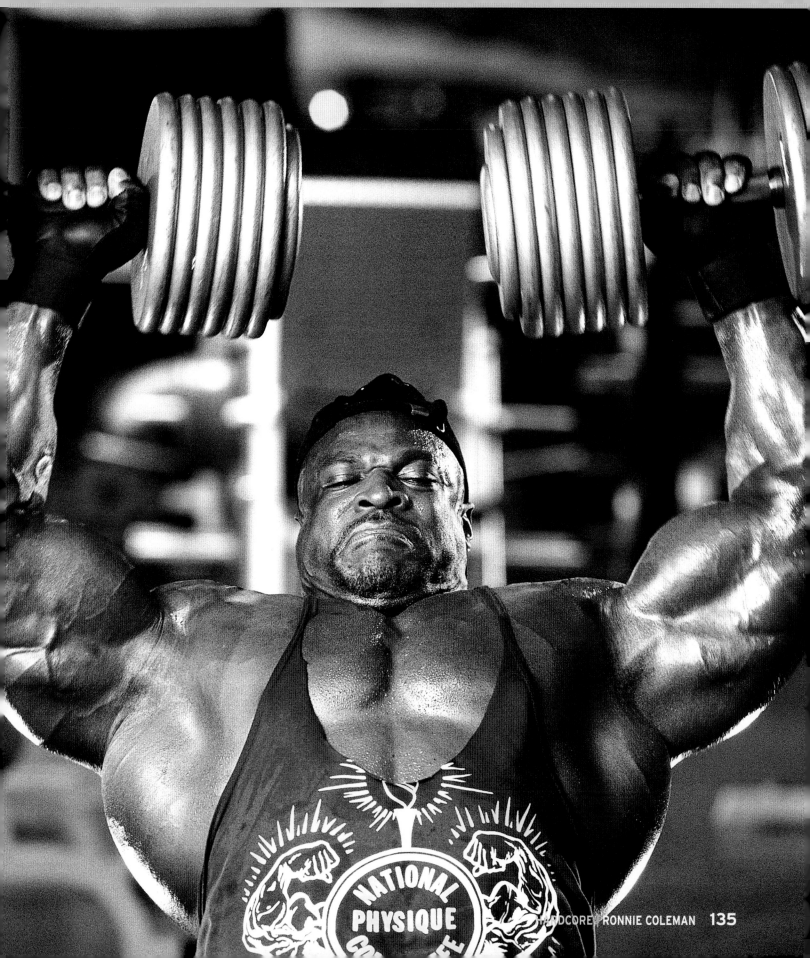

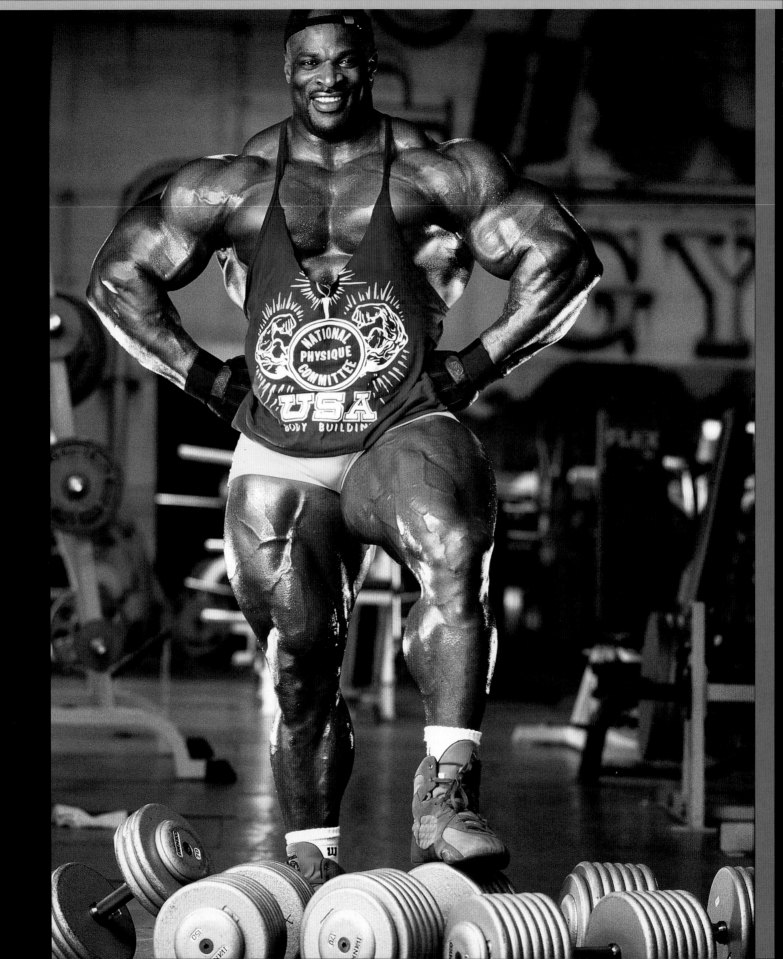

DAY 4 - THURSDAY
Workout B: Back, Biceps, Delts

BACK

EXERCISE	SETS
T-Bar Row	4
One-Arm Dumbbell Row	4
Wide-Grip Pull-Up	3
Pulldown to Front (or) Close-Grip Row	3

BICEPS

EXERCISE	SETS
Alternating Dumbbell Curl	4
EZ-Bar Preacher Curl	3
One-Arm Cable Curl	3
Dumbbell Concentration Curl	3

DELTS

EXERCISE	SETS
Smith-Machine Press	4
Dumbbell Lateral Raise (drop sets)	2 (20/15/10/8 reps per set)
Dumbbell Front Raise	3
Bent-Over Lateral Raise	3

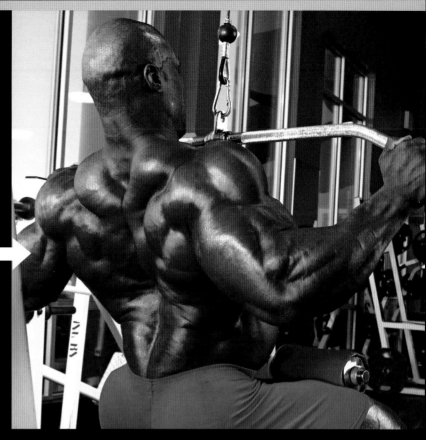

DAY 5 - FRIDAY
Workout B: Legs

THIGHS

EXERCISE	SETS
Leg Extension	4 (15-30 reps)
Front Barbell Squat	5
Hack Squat	3
Romanian Deadlift	3
Seated Leg Curl	3

CALVES

Standing Calf Raise	4
Seated Calf Raise	4

DAY 6 - SATURDAY
Workout B: Chest, Triceps

CHEST

EXERCISE	SETS
Incline Dumbbell Press	4
Flat-Bench Dumbbell Press	3
Decline Dumbbell Press	3
Flat-Bench Dumbbell Flye	3

TRICEPS

EXERCISE	SETS
Close-Grip Bench Press	4
Lying French Press	3
Dumbbell Kickback	3

FOUR TIMES PER WEEK
(At the end of any workout)

ABS

EXERCISE	SETS
Crunch	3 (to failure)

CHAPTER 9
NUTRITION
& SUPPLEMENTS

Nutrition is vital to success — I can't stress that point enough. So many people go to the gym and toil for months, even years, wondering why they never see any appreciable gains. If this is you, you probably need look no further than your eating habits.

Building a body is like building a house. You can go through the motions all you want on the construction site, hammering and sawing, but if you don't have any building blocks to work with in the first place, you will end up with nothing. No lumber, no house. No clean sources of protein and carbohydrates, no body. Yes, it's that simple.

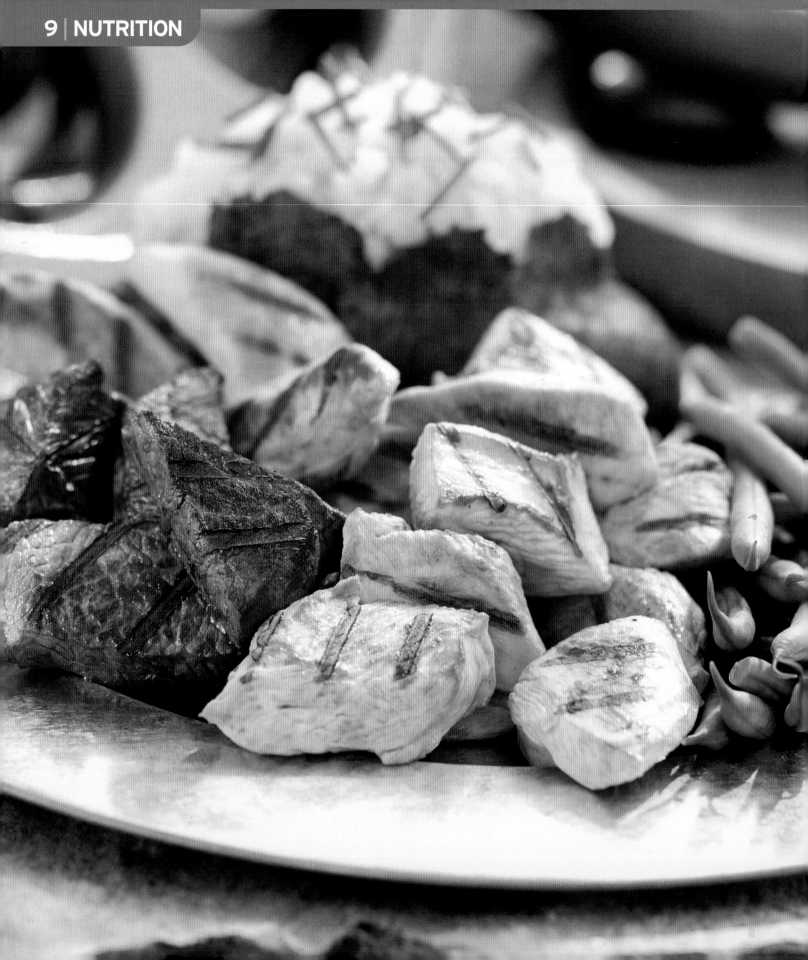

OFF-SEASON: GAINING MASS

When you're bulking up, nutrition can prove to be more challenging than training — when you train, you only need to focus for 90 minutes. To stay the course and eat enough to grow, you need to concentrate every waking hour.

Overall, I'd say diet is about 70% of the mass-building equation when compared with training. The plain and simple truth is that if you don't pay attention to what you put in your mouth, you'll never achieve the look of a bodybuilder. You still have to train, but I think dieting is harder because it requires more mental focus.

In mass mode, I eat a minimum of 5–6 times a day. When I first started getting serious about growing, my philosophy was eat until I was full, then come back and eat again soon after. These days my diet has a little more nuance than that, but the core is the same: To grow, you have to make yourself eat at regular intervals, whether you feel hungry or not.

As I show you what I do, remember that this is the diet of a full-time bodybuilder. This is my job — most people may not want to go to these extremes. It means nights out, and eating whatever you want, is rare rather than the norm. It means preparing meals ahead of time, and sticking with staples such as chicken breasts and protein shakes no matter how tired you get of them. I do it because it's how I make my living: Food is not enjoyment for me; it's part of the process by which I survive. Just keep that in mind as you read on.

For my protein, my primary sources are beef, turkey and chicken. On the carb side, I have grits, pancakes and baked potatoes. I'm not a big fan of vegetables, but they're a good source of fiber. If you can stomach them, you should try to have a vegetable with at least three of your meals.

Here's an example of a typical off-season day; my food choices won't be the exact same every day, but this gives you an idea of how a meal might look, as well as my totals for the day. I'll eat these meals spaced 2½–3 hours apart.

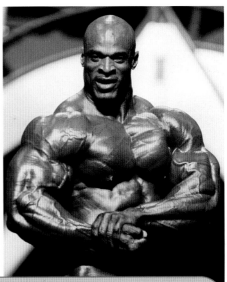

	FOOD	CALORIES	PROTEIN (g)	CARBS (g)	FAT (g)
MEAL 1	1 tall stack pancakes	896	24	170	12
	or 2 cups grits	322	6	64	4
	Protein shake	330	60	9	5
MEAL 2	14-oz. chicken breast	660	124	0	14
	4 cups white rice	820	20	180	2
MEAL 3	5 oz. top round steak broiled (precooked weight)	335	44	0	17
	Large baked potato	252	7	56	trace
MEAL 4	Meal replacement shake	580	90	36	9
MEAL 5	2 chicken sandwiches:				
	2 7-oz. chicken breasts	660	124	0	14
	2 hamburger buns	260	10	44	5
	Swiss cheese (2 slices each)	320	24	0	24
	1 glass lemonade	134	trace	34	trace
MEAL 6	Meal replacement shake	580	90	36	9
	Fruit	216	trace	114	trace
TOTALS		6,365	623	743	115

I try to eat a meal high in protein and complex carbs about an hour and a half before I work out. I'm not overly concerned about post-workout nutrition until contest prep. In the 12 weeks leading up to a show, I'll have some chicken and rice right after I train.

Having seen the sample diet day on the previous page, you may ask, "Ronnie, do you ever have cheat meals or cheat days in the off-season?" In a word, yes. I try to eat clean most of the time, but I think you have to cheat now and then to give your body a jolt. If you're hungry or if you have a craving that just won't quit, you should indulge that impulse on occasion. If you don't, the craving will just get worse and you may totally blow your diet. There's nothing wrong with cheating in the off-season, as long as it doesn't become a daily (or hourly) occurrence.

PRECONTEST: GETTING SHREDDED

As I transition into precontest mode, you'll notice that my diet isn't that much different from my off-season diet. In the past, my off-season eating plan was often a "no rules" scenario — pizza, hamburgers, cheesecake, pretty much anything I wanted — but I've gotten more disciplined year-round. And the results have been amazing: I came to the 2003 Olympia stage at a huge and shredded all-time best of 287 pounds, a full 37 pounds heavier than the year before. It also may just be age; when you're young, your body can overcome a lot, but now I'm 40, and although I have no doubt you can compete successfully in bodybuilding at 40

and beyond, you need to be a heck of a lot more disciplined in your approach.

In precontest mode, there are three rules: Eat extremely clean, eat at regular intervals, and maintain your protein intake at off-season levels. You make your manipulations to carbs and fat, but protein is necessary, especially for me because I don't back off my training intensity one inch. I want to build muscle right up to the very day of the contest. I also cut out red meat from my diet in the final 12 weeks.

At the 1997 Mr. Olympia, the year before I first won, I learned a valuable lesson: continue my off-season diet as long as possible. That year, I started my contest diet 16 weeks out, and it screwed me up completely; I ended up in ninth place. It was far too long to diet. Now from week 16 to week 12, I don't really deprive myself of anything, but merely ease myself into a diet mode. Then, when I'm 12 weeks out from the show, my official precontest diet, which is encapsulated below, begins.

DIET IS ABOUT 70% OF THE MASS-BUILDING EQUATION

	FOOD	CALORIES	PROTEIN (g)	CARBS (g)	FAT (g)
MEAL 1	2 cups grits	322	6	64	4
	Protein shake	330	60	9	5
MEAL 2	14-oz. chicken breast	660	124	0	14
	8-oz. baked potato	168	4	37	trace
MEAL 3	14-oz. chicken breast	660	124	0	14
	2 cups white rice	410	5	45	trace
MEAL 4	14-oz. turkey breast	540	120	0	3
	8-oz. baked potato	168	4	37	trace
MEAL 5	14-oz. chicken breast	660	124	0	14
	2 cups white rice	410	5	45	trace
BEFORE BED MEAL 6	Protein shake	330	60	9	5
TOTALS		4,658	636	246	59

Note: Protein shakes are mixed with water. You can add ice cubes to give texture.

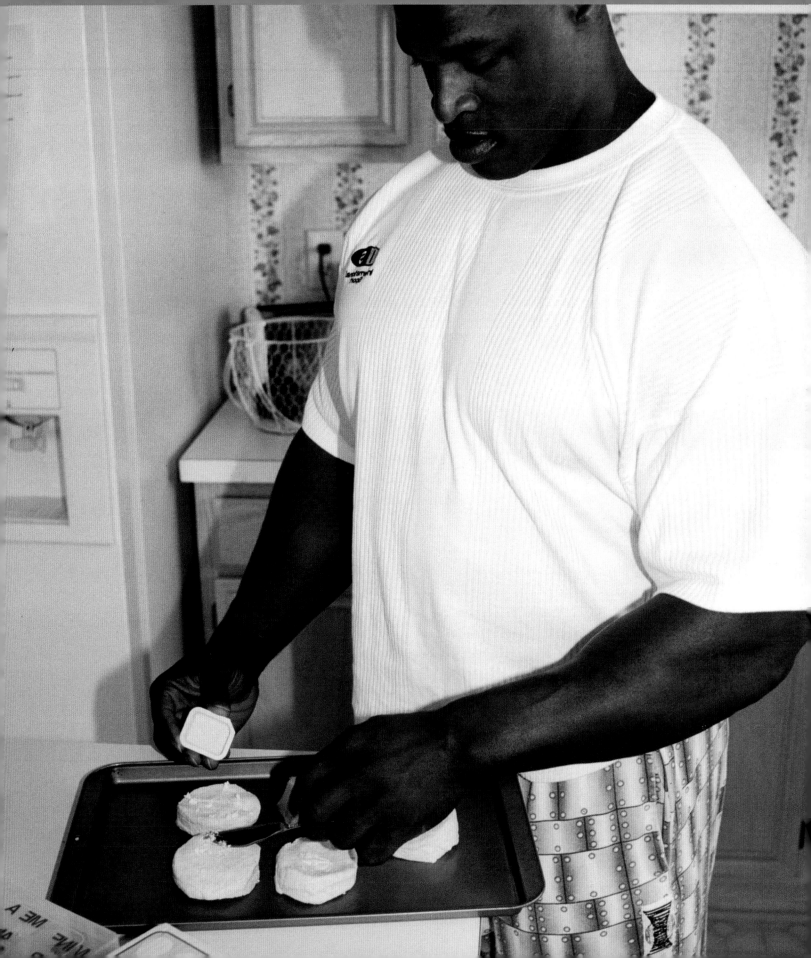

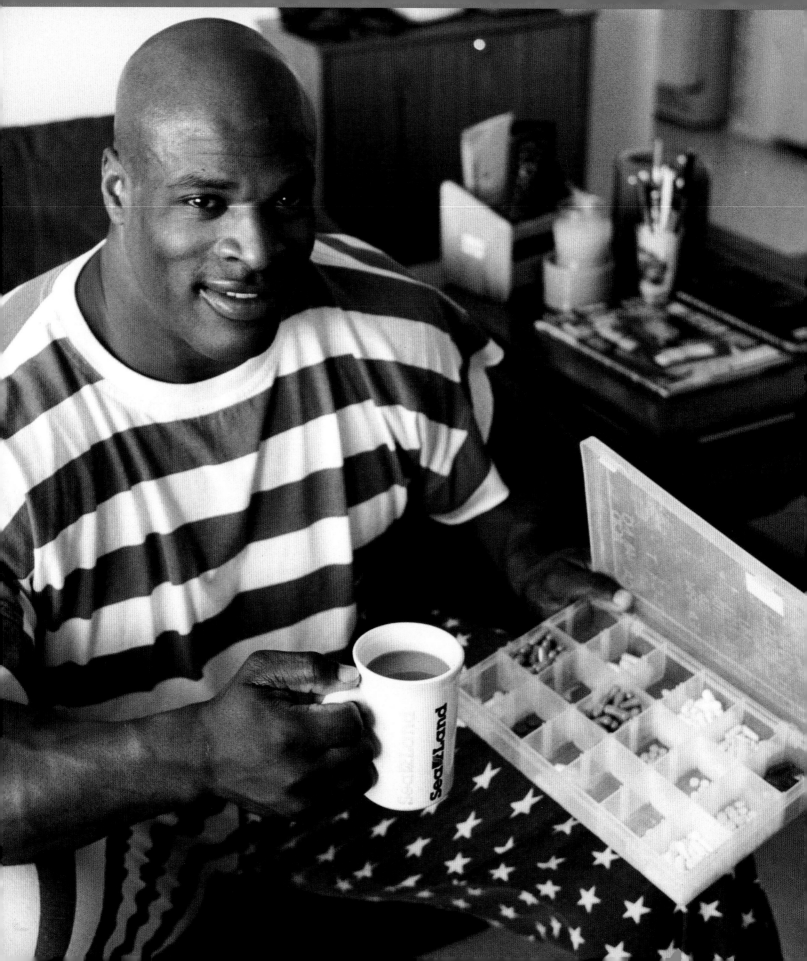

In addition to allowing me to maintain mass, these meals also facilitate the stabilization of my diet. Since my carbs are subordinated to my protein and since they are held constant for the duration of my contest-prep period, they're easy to control. I know they aren't going to spill over or drop to a depletion level.

Actually, I'm not so regimented that I'll allow my body to become so accustomed to my diet that it will stop responding favorably to chicken, turkey, potatoes, rice and the protein drinks. I occasionally "shock" it; I will go for three-day periods during which my first three meals of the day will be of the normal protein-carb combinations, but then I'll drop carbs for the last three. I'm tricking my body.

Of course, it's necessary to keep an eye on how I appear in the mirror and manipulate my carbs up or down accordingly; everyone responds a little differently to food and macronutrients, so you need to learn how to notice the effects as you experiment. If you're a serious bodybuilder and your goal is to step onstage, you should go the extra step and keep a detailed log, so over time you have a blueprint for what works and what doesn't.

Six weeks out, I add a second one-hour cardio session each day. A week before the show, I start carb depleting. If the contest is on a Saturday, I drop down to 100 grams of carbs on the previous Sunday, Monday and Tuesday, then carb load on Wednesday and Thursday, taking it really high, as much as 600 grams, even to the point where I'm spilling over a little bit. On Friday, I go back down low, maybe to about 300 grams, or whatever is needed for fine-tuning.

The inability to hold your peak comes from either deprivation or complication, or a combination thereof, so keep it elementary. Make protein the basis of your precontest or "getting cut" diet, and everything else will fall in line.

A WORD ON SUPPLEMENTS

Here's my take on supplements: Yes, I use them and with great success. But don't let them become the centerpiece of your bodybuilding approach. I know it happens to a lot of people out there. I remember a letter I received from a fan once. Take a look at his regimen:

"I use aminos, protein shakes, glutamine, and I cycle creatine into my diet, six weeks on and six weeks off. Of course, I take multivitamins and minerals. I also take extra Vitamin C, calcium, magnesium, etc. because there's not enough in any multivitamin. My vitamin carrier is a small tackle box from Wal-Mart. I never leave home without it."

The advice I offered to him? Turn your tackle box upside down, refill it with freshwater spinner lures and light-test trolling line, then go fishing. You need a rest from your obsession with supplements.

I've said it before and I'll say it again: Supplements are just that. They're not intended to replace your training and diet, but rather, to augment them. Good training and good food come first. Those two alone are the foundation on which everything else in bodybuilding is built.

You should consider taking vitamins, minerals and other supplements only when your training and diet are in place. But don't go crazy with supplementation. Stay away from the "supplements-are-everything" mindset, like the guy in the above example.

Now, with that warning, I will tell you that I take a variety of supplements year-round, including creatine, glutamine, a multivitamin/mineral, and extra doses of Vitamins C and E. As you saw in my off-season and precontest diets, I also make ample use of protein powders and meal-replacement shakes. But all of this is supplemental to my regular diet. When the cornerstones of bodybuilding progress — intense workouts backed up by a good diet — are in place, supplements can give you an added boost.

Okay, I've given you my training and my diet programs. In the next chapter, I answer some of the more common questions I get. Those answers should help you fill in the blanks and put the final pieces together as you devise your own plan for bodybuilding success.

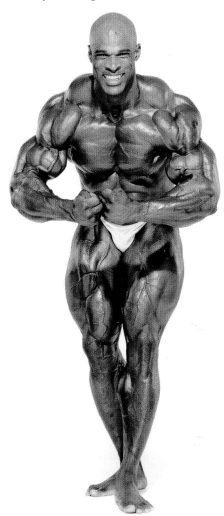

CHAPTER 10

Q&A WITH THE CHAMP

No matter where I travel in the United States or across the globe, I get a lot of the same questions from fans. From training to nutrition to everything in between, people want to know what it takes, and what they need to do, to gain strength and build muscle without packing on fat. Fitness isn't just a phenomenon of the U.S. – it is truly a global pursuit. In this chapter, I'll cover some common questions I'm asked: How can I get rock-hard abs faster? How can I overcome injuries, and avoid them in the first place? What can I do to bench more? How can I get that super-hard look of the pros? What can I do to keep my motivation and intensity sky-high month after month, year after year? All of those answers, and more, are here.

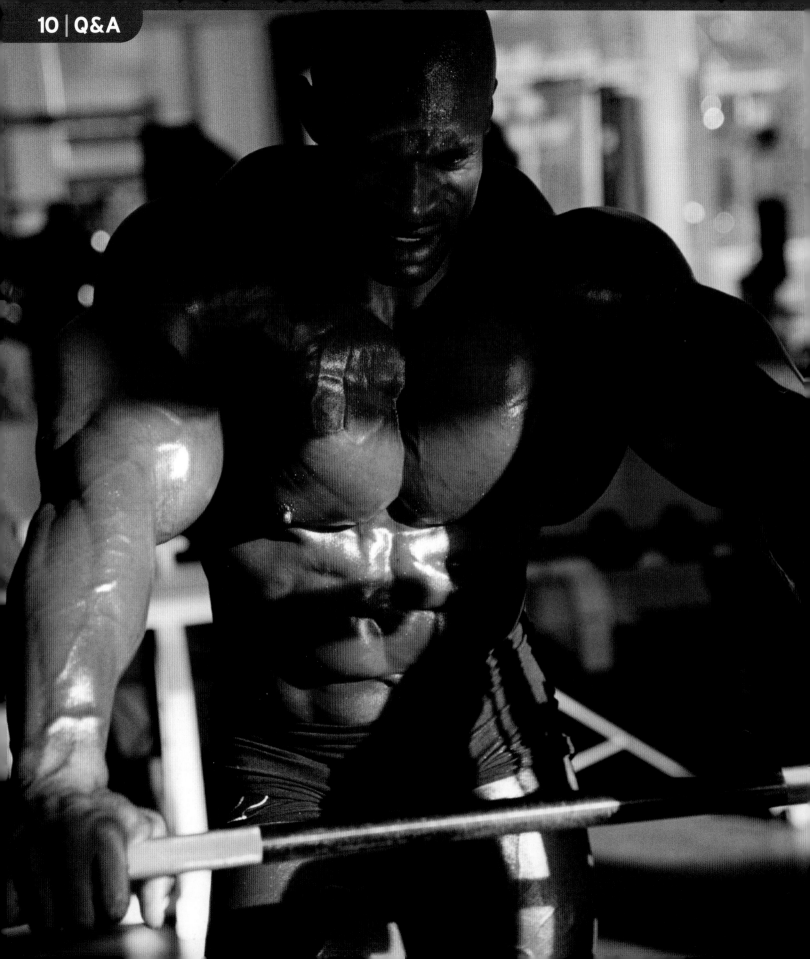

ON FAILURE VS. FATIGUE...

What is your theory on "going to failure" in your workouts?

First, you need to know there's "going to failure," and then there's the concept of wholly fatiguing your muscles. They're both different, and you need to do both. If you "go to failure," it means you can't get another repetition on a given set. If you "totally fatigue a muscle," it means the muscle will no longer fire.

The two are similar in the sense that they both imply having reached a limit, but they are different limits. Failure is functional, fatigue is physiological. Failure has more to do with what's outside your body, fatigue has more to do with what's inside your body. Failure has more to do with an individual muscle, fatigue has more to do with a complete bodypart.

Most important, going to failure doesn't mean you have totally fatigued the muscle you're working. It only means that all of the multiple biomechanical systems, muscles and leverages involved in performing that movement are weakened to the point at which you can no longer lift the weight. It doesn't necessarily mean that any of those individual muscles has been totally fatigued.

Grasping this concept is crucial for bodybuilders because it's possible to take every exercise to failure for the rest of your life and still not build appreciable muscle mass. You'll build strength, to be sure, because you're dividing the growth that occurs from your weight training among various muscle groups and improving their collective ability to lift that weight. The growth of the individual muscles

in those muscle groups may be minimal in some cases, however, because you'll reach failure in your ability to perform the exercise before any of those individual muscles has a chance to be worked to its limit, or completely fatigued.

The modern approach of progressive weight training, in which we start a bodypart workout with compound movements and finish with isolation movements, is intended to cover both failure and fatigue, thereby promoting both strength and muscle growth from the very same workout. The initial compound exercise, taken to failure, builds overall strength in the bodypart and parcels out the resulting muscle growth among all the areas of that particular bodypart. Compound bodypart "failure" exercises thus give us overall mass.

After failure of a bodypart is reached with a compound movement, we then focus on individual muscles in that bodypart. We do this by

exercises. That leads us to two other essential terms: "proper performance of an exercise" and "intensity."

Too often it's assumed that proper performance of an exercise is important only for isolation exercises. Not so. Without proper performance, failure, too, will suffer. If you're sloppy and cheat by swinging the weight with bodyparts other than the one you're trying to work, they will reach failure before the intended bodypart, and nothing will benefit from the exercise. In this regard, proper performance of an exercise may actually be more important for compound movements than for isolation movements.

The same consequence comes from not applying maximum intensity to every set. Intensity is a focusing of maximum effort, and it's the only way to fatigue all fibers of a muscle. Fatigue, then, takes over where failure leaves off: Once you reach failure, you keep on going with isolation movements until you reach total

UNDERSTANDING "FAILURE" VS. "FATIGUE" CAN MAKE A HUGE DIFFERENCE IN YOUR QUEST FOR MORE MUSCLE

applying isolation exercises, which are intended to take each individual muscle the rest of the way to fatigue and enable it to grow independently of the rest of the bodypart. This is where we get the term "muscle separation."

The point so far is to warn you not to mistake failure for fatigue. Obviously, we need both, but whether we attain both is contingent upon getting the most out of their relative

fatigue. That's the purpose of forced reps, for example: They liberate you from the limitations of bodypart failure, so you can keep pumping ntil every fiber of that muscle is devastated and will no longer fire.

For me, the rep ranges that work best for taking a muscle to failure and beyond to total fatigue are 10-15. I advise that you try the same. Just remember, when you reach failure, your workout has only begun.

PYRAMIDING FOR GROWTH...

Can you explain the concept of pyramiding up your weight during an exercise?

In pyramid training, you progressively increase the poundage you lift with each successive set (i.e., your first set might be 50 pounds, the second 75, the third 100, etc., all the way to your maximum poundage for that particular exercise). This is done to ensure safety. If you lifted the maximum poundage on your first set, you'd probably injure yourself because the bodypart involved wouldn't be warmed up, nor would your muscles have had time to coordinate their tensions in order to handle that amount of weight. After all, those coordinated tensions change with every change in the weight, which means that the greater the differential, the more shock it is to the muscles. (The smaller increments you use for pyramiding, the safer. You'll also find that a small increase gives you more ability to properly handle the next heavier set.)

Some bodybuilders pyramid their repetitions in terms of percentage of failure. For the first set, the repetitions may be to only 60% of failure, the second set to 75% of failure, the third set to 80%, etc., until on the last set, they go all the way to 100% failure with their repetitions.

Many bodybuilders use the increasing-percentage-of-failure technique for their repetitions while still incrementally decreasing their reps as they pyramid the weight. Others use the increasing-percentage-of-failure technique and keep their reps constant through all sets as they pyramid the weight. Still others go to failure on every set, but they add enough weight so that their repetitions also progressively decrease each time.

What works best for me is to keep my repetitions constant as I pyramid the weight for each set, going to failure every time by varying the pace of the repetitions — very slow contractions for light sets and proportionately faster ones for heavier sets. Almost every exercise I do for each bodypart gets 3–4 sets of 10–15 repetitions each. However, that's far from the complete story, because the most intricate program of pyramid training sets in the world won't put you a step closer to success unless you perform each repetition to perfection.

Your workout isn't about how much you pyramid, nor is it about how often you rep to failure; it's about controlling the weights so that each muscle is contracted properly. All of the variations I described will work if you think about your muscle moving the weight; but all of the techniques, even my own, will be worthless if you think fancy-sounding training principles alone are all you need.

THE SECRET TO AB TRAINING...

I'd really like to get a six-pack. What can I do to accelerate my progress in my ab-training regimen?

A chain is only as strong as its weakest link, and the same principle applies to your body. If you want strong and muscular abs, the rest of your bodyparts must also be strong and muscular. No muscle in your body functions properly all by itself. Think about what your abdominals do: they connect your upper body to your lower body. Without your abs, you would be walking around with your torso slumped over between your legs and your head dragging on the ground. Your abs also work in conjunction with your back, leg, shoulder and hip muscles. If you had only abdominals but not those other muscles, your body would flop over backwards, your spine would collapse and rupture all of its discs, and you wouldn't be able to stand upright, let alone walk or lift anything.

As bodybuilders, even though we train bodyparts separately, the lifting is never truly done by that bodypart alone. The abs are almost always involved — or at least they should be. With pressing exercises for your chest, your abs tighten to stabilize your upper and lower body. Heavy biceps curls rely on strong abs to keep your body upright, so you can concentrate the force within your biceps and achieve a full range of motion. For deadlifts and squats, abdominal strength is just as important for stabilizing your body as back and leg strength is for the lift itself.

Conversely, you can't properly train your abs without bringing your hip flexors, spinal erectors and glutes into play. All of those muscle groups need to tighten as one in what's called a "compound" manner. If they don't, your pelvis will rotate forward against the base of your spine, which not only prevents you from getting a full contraction of your abs but also compresses your vertebrae. All the more reason, then, to work your abs more for strength than for appearance. Aim for the former goal, and you get both; aim for the latter, and you'll end up with neither.

The more compound exercises you do for other bodyparts, the better abs you'll have, because they'll be required to do more work. Keep in mind, however, that your abs become involved only if you use basic free-weight exercises that require your abdominals to provide a

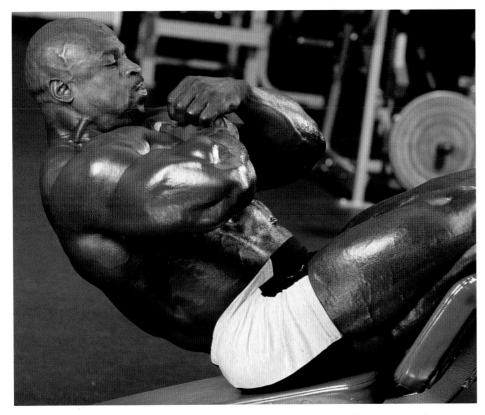

tight connection between your upper and lower body. For chest, that means flat and incline barbell or dumbbell presses, although cable crossovers also require a lot of abdominal tension. For biceps, any heavy standing barbell or dumbbell curl requires intense abdominal contractions for stability, as do standing french presses or overhead extensions for triceps. Nearly any free-weight shoulder exercise, particularly military presses and standing or seated dumbbell raises, benefits your abs. For back, you can't do deadlifts or barbell rows without first contracting your abs as hard as you can. And any pro will tell you the procedure for squatting is to tighten your abs to relieve pressure from your spine, flex your traps to get the bar up and off your deltoids, squeeze your hips so they provide a foundation for your torso, then maintain all of that as you squat.

Of course, you should also work your abs specifically. I often use crunches, decline crunches and hanging leg raises myself, but whatever ab exercise you do,

always make sure the exercise shortens the distance between your sternum and your pelvis — if it doesn't, your abs aren't flexing and extending through their intended range of motion. Never arch backwards or keep your torso straight.

Incorporate these tips, but never lose sight of the basic principles for achieving the best abdominals possible: proper diet; years of hard, consistent training; and a balanced, heavy, free-weight workout utilizing basic exercises that combine different bodyparts held together by your abdominals.

ON PAIN...

What can I do to mini-mize post-workout muscle soreness?

Pain is as much a part of a bodybuilder's life as skinless chicken breasts. A bodybuilder judges the effectiveness of his workouts by how far into the future

his pump pains him. Of course, that depends on your ability to distinguish between bad (injury) pain and good (pump) pain. You should easily tell the difference: Bad pain severely restricts your poundages the next time you lift. With good pain, you can still lift your max at the next session.

Before we go any further, here's a fact of life all lifters must face. You need several years of consistent training to condition and build your muscles so they can handle hard workouts that give you a good pump without debilitating soreness. With persistence, you'll reach that level. At this point in my career, I train harder, heavier and more often than ever, yet I no longer become sore or stiff or even develop a burn. I do, however, get a great pump every time.

One cause of soreness is not training often enough. If you take too much time off between workouts, your muscles lose their conditioning so when you hit them hard again, it's equivalent to starting over. The lactic-acid buildup and resulting soreness will be greater than in a conditioned muscle that has been trained more frequently.

Hard-trained muscle needs rest, but most bodybuilders use that principle as an excuse. The maximum amount of time between workouts for the same bodypart should be a week, but I prefer less. You should also get in at least four days a week of good hard training; again, I prefer more. The only way to reduce soreness and stiffness is to condition your body, but you can't just wait for your body to become conditioned; you have to force it to become conditioned. You have to push it past the pain barrier, just as you have to push yourself past the psychological barrier that you think is pain but is actually the greatest reward awaiting a bodybuilder: a blood-swelling, pressure-packed, muscle-popping pump.

ON INJURIES...

Have you ever had an injury that made you stop training? If so, what was it, and what did you do for it?

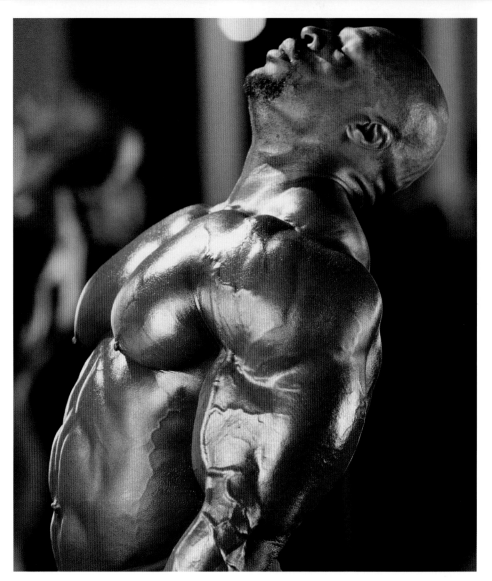

You should instead ask me which injury I suffered today. It seems as though I pull or tear something every time I set foot in the gym. I have injuries year-round — it's been that way since I started — but at least that means I'm pushing myself to improve. A human being can't possibly bodybuild correctly without getting injured sometimes. You learn your lesson about what you did wrong, work around it and do the best you can.

I once hurt my knee so badly that I thought I'd broken my kneecap. Fortunately, X-rays showed that it was only a severe strain. When I returned to the gym, I simply lightened up the weight and started over. That did the trick. Eventually, I was back up to my normal poundage.

Years ago, I ruptured a disc doing squats and couldn't train for two weeks — I could barely walk. It took me a full year to get back up to my normal 600 pounds for 10-12 reps. My back still bothers me sometimes, but I do what I can. That's the essence of our sport. During any of these injuries, did I ever once consider quitting bodybuilding? Never. No matter which bodypart was injured, I continued training all the others, and along the way learned the lesson that bodybuilding should be more about character building than bodybuilding. It really is about doing what you can in the face of adversity and disappointment. It's about exploring your limits and learning that as a human being, you have some. More important, it's about learning that those limits are put there to make you better, to put some starch in your spine, and to teach you how to navigate through life. It's about growing up.

The Mr. Olympia title, to me, has never been about having the best body in the world. That's only the result of continually trying to make myself better in every way, regardless of circumstances. I've always claimed that if I lost two limbs, I could still improve the two that remained; if I lost all of them, I could still improve my torso. In so doing, I'd be a bigger man than the guy who looks in the mirror and swoons from his own perfection.

Always go for progress, not perfection. The latter is not only a dream but also a dead end. Even if you could attain perfection, your joy would end because you could never improve on it. You would have to "settle" for perfection. Fulfillment, on the other hand, results from having overcome adversity by determined, daily accomplishments, step-by-step improvements that never end. In never ending, they never stop satisfying. Perfection denies us that opportunity.

Every time I have another injury, I give thanks, because it makes me wiser and stronger. I suggest you do the same. No matter what injuries you face now or in the future, I guarantee you this: Keep training as best you can, and you'll be a bigger man than ever.

ON STAYING THE COURSE...

How are you able to stick with your off-season program during your precontest prep, while other bodybuilders ditch heavy strength training in favor of lighter weights and higher reps in the 15–30 range?

The purpose of a precontest period is to make your muscularity as visible as possible. That means getting your bodyfat as low as possible and your muscles as big as possible. Contrary to popular misconception, the two are not incompatible.

Prevailing myths hold that "as you lose weight, you lose a lot of strength" and "higher reps burn more calories," but I think those are cop-outs by underachievers who use contest prep as a vacation. To me, contest prep is just the opposite: a moment of truth, a trial by fire.

If I can do it, you can, too. By reducing your bodyfat, you increase your body's muscle-to-fat ratio. Since you then have more muscle relative to the weight you're lugging around all day, you'll have more endurance, intensity and comparative strength.

Continue training with your heaviest weights, and you'll burn more calories than if you use lighter weights with higher reps. Heavy weight makes you exert more energy, use more muscles, work each muscle deeper and fatigue the muscles to a greater deficit. With higher reps, even in prolonged sets, the total calories burned will still come up short, compared with a heavy maximum-intensity workout.

Unfortunately, many bodybuilders are in worse condition — small, wan, drawn and exhausted — before a contest than when they're not competing because they back off from everything that made them massive and cut in the first place, namely, power-packed food and heavy, intense training.

Don't reduce the muscle-building nutrients in your diet precontest. Maintain or increase your protein intake, and find the calorie level that supplies you with enough energy to sustain your customarily furious workouts, while allowing you to gradually burn excess bodyfat without burning muscle. Break down your total consumption into six meals a day, but have a sufficient portion of protein in each of them. (To accelerate bodyfat loss, I have chicken or turkey, but that's because I don't like fish. In meals one and six, I substitute a protein shake. The rest of the food choices are baked potatoes, rice and grits.)

People still have a hard time believing that I still use the same slate of exercises and set and rep schemes I had years ago, but it's absolutely true. The only real difference is in the weights. I'm stronger now, so I can lift more. That's the only change I make, and I recommend the same for you. Once you've settled on a general scheme that gives you the best muscle growth for a bodypart, stay with it and try to gradually increase the weight you use.

ON STICKING POINTS...

I'm stuck at 225 on my bench press. How can I get past this plateau?

Sticking points, cessation of gains or any other form of "hitting the wall" happens to every bodybuilder at some point and, if you're not prepared, can be demoralizing. That, however, is the only bad news. The good news is that it's your opportunity to learn the art and science of troubleshooting, which we all must master if we expect to make it through life.

Here's how you should approach that sticking point. First, make sure you have a realistic perspective. Is your reach beyond your grasp when it comes to the poundage you're trying to lift? When it's not coming easy, take advantage of the smallest increments — if you can do 225, but want to progress beyond that, your next increment should be no more than 230 if you're struggling.

Your problem could be one of technique as well. Maybe you're not executing the movement properly. The first hint of this might be revealed in a visual assessment of your physique. Look at your deltoids. Are they proportionately more developed than your pecs? If they are, it's likely that you're pressing more with your shoulders than your chest.

Your chest is one of those bodyparts that's best fatigued by movements that are assisted by other bodyparts — incline, decline and flat-bench presses are the best moves for chest, but your delts and triceps will come into play on any press. The only way you can contract your pecs effectively is by means of your lats (which "open" and "close" your pecs), your traps and rhomboids (which prevent your body's center of gravity from shifting into your shoulder girdle), your abs (which stabilize your torso), and your lower body (which prevents your entire body from sliding downward and keeps the responsibility for the press in your pecs).

Now try bench pressing again, but this time put your whole body into it. Think in terms of doing whatever it takes to press that barbell up, not in terms of "feeling" your pecs getting pumped (that comes from other isolation-type exercises later in a chest workout). Plant your feet firmly, and be prepared to press with your legs so your entire torso cocks itself like a spring, nice and tight. Grip the bar hard and as you lower it, tighten your body and squeeze your lats together, bringing your chest up to meet the bar. As you press, squeeze your pecs together by flaring your lats.

If your bench-pressing problem is traceable to poor technique, this aggressive approach should yield an immediate improvement. If it doesn't, the next troubleshooting step is to see if you're overtraining or undertraining the bodypart. Here's a rule of thumb: More than three times a week is overtraining; once a week is undertraining. Further, more than 25 total sets per bodypart is overtraining; less than 15 is undertraining.

Prioritize your chest workout so that it falls after a rest day. Your first exercise should be bench presses. Pyramid up through seven all-out working sets, starting at 15 reps, to 12, 10, 8, 6, 5 and maxing out at 3 reps for your seventh set.

If this still doesn't work, then your problem could be the selection of exercises in your chest workout. Reorient them to the following all-power movements: bench presses, incline barbell presses, flat-bench dumbbell presses and superset incline dumbbell presses with flat-bench dumbbell flyes to finish. Stay with seven working sets for bench presses and use four working sets of five reps for each of the other exercises.

If all of this fails, which I can't believe is possible, the final troubleshooting step has to lie in your confidence: There could be no other conclusion than you're afraid of that barbell above you. If so, use a spotter (as you should always while benching) while you explore your outer limits and get comfortable with a big weight in your hands. That intangible quality of confidence will do more for your progress than all of the bodybuilding science I can provide.

ON PULLING STRENGTH...
How can I get stronger in the pull-up?

First, let's set the table: For the sake of this book, a pull-up and a chin-up are almost the same animal. A pull-up is performed with your palms facing forward; a chin-up is performed with your palms facing toward you. You can vary the width of your grip on the bar with either exercise. Going wider puts more emphasis on the lats, coming in closer exerts more biceps in the pull.

Chinning and pull-up power is a product of the combined strength of several different muscle groups: lats, biceps, forearms, rear delts, upper back, chest — not to mention other body-stabilizing muscles like the abs. Here are three of the best exercises to strengthen all of these elements, giving you more punch in your pull.

(1) WIDE-GRIP PULL-UP: This movement is essential for building into your back the squeezing power your upper and lower lats need to hoist your body upward. Reach up and, using an overhand grip, grasp an overhead bar approximately 6–8 inches beyond shoulder width. Start the movement with your body hanging at a full stretch, then pull yourself up until your chin is level with the bar. Lower slowly to a full stretch, and repeat. Keep your lats and the movement tight and smooth to avoid swinging.

To develop your hand and forearm strength, alternate with a thumbs-around-the-bar (normal) grip one workout and a thumbs-over-the-bar, so your fingers and thumb are all on the same side, the next. When you're able to complete 12 reps, strap a weight belt with a 25-pound plate around your waist, and again work up to 12 reps. Continue this process of increasing poundage month to month. Do four sets total as a part of your back workout.

(2) BEHIND-THE-NECK PULL-UP: This exercise is hard to beat for developing strength in your upper lats, rear delts, upper back and rhomboids — all of which are crucial for getting those final couple of inches of pull at the top. Use the same grip as with wide-grip pull-ups, except keep your thumbs over the bar instead of wrapped around it to allow for a higher pull. Get a full stretch at the bottom, then squeeze your lats to get as high as possible, bringing your head in front of the bar. Try to touch the bar to the base of your neck. Keep the move tight, avoiding swinging at all costs. Do four sets, and use the same repetition scheme and weight-belt additions as with the wide-grip pull-up.

(3) WEIGHTED CHIN-UP: This exercise is hard to beat for building size and strength in the back and biceps. Use an underhand grip, palms facing you, with your hands at outer-chest width on the bar. Get a full stretch at the bottom, then pull yourself as high as possible, bringing your chin above the level of the bar. Lower yourself slowly. Do four sets, and use the same repetition scheme and weight-belt additions as with the two previous exercises.

To incorporate these three moves into your training, do the first two exercises — wide-grip pull-ups and behind-the-neck pull-ups — in the same workout with your other back training. (If you follow my workout on page 17, do 2 sets of wide-grip pull-ups instead of 3 and add 2 sets behind-the-neck.) Do weighted chins at least once per week on a separate day, at least 1–2 days after your back session. Before you know it, you'll be chinning like a Marine.

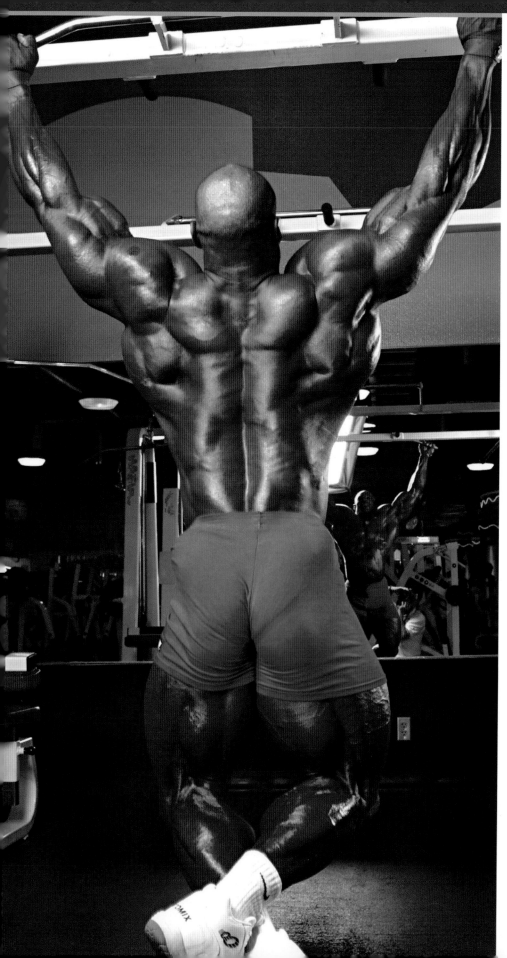

ON SIZE...

I want to compete in my first bodybuilding show. Should building mass be my No. 1 priority at this stage?

Bodybuilding isn't just about being the biggest guy onstage. I had a friend who, because he was the biggest guy walking into a particular contest, thought he would win easily. But that didn't happen — in a lineup of much less massive but harder, more defined bodybuilders, he faded into the background and didn't even appear to be that muscular.

Yes, I realize that I am the biggest Mr. Olympia champion to date, but I would still argue that my mass alone isn't the reason for my Sandow-winning success. Bodybuilding doesn't mean just building mass. It's about symmetry, proportion, definition, size, fullness and complete development of all bodyparts. It requires a dual approach of increasing overall mass, as distinct from increasing individual muscle size, and dieting away interstitial fat to show separation between individual muscles.

To steadily increase mass while pursuing those other goals, I would recommend training with heavy basic exercises right up to the show. Stay within a 10–15 rep range. That's what I do. I don't make any major changes as I'm getting closer to a contest, but rather I stick to the same formula, off-season and on. My bench press, for example, may be 135 for 20 reps, 225 for 15, 315 for another 15 and finally 405 for 12, whether I'm deep in off-season mode or three weeks out from competing. I'm constantly pushing my body to grow, and backing off won't give my body the impetus it needs to do so.

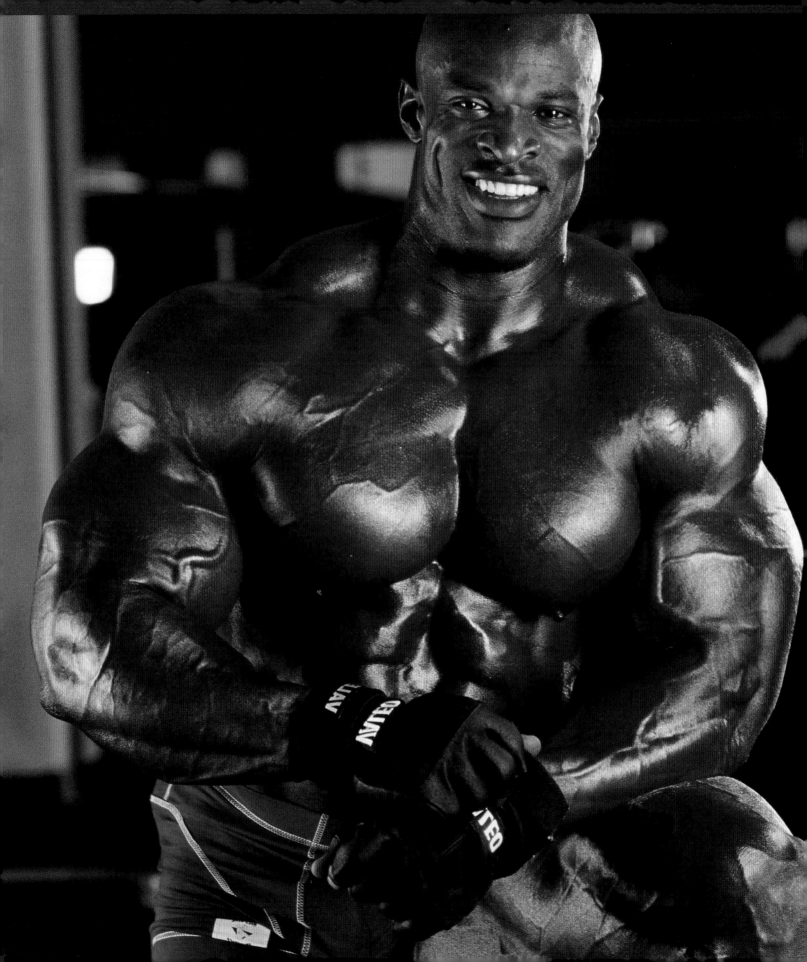

Having said that, there is a time in the week before a show that I do back off a little. In that week, I lower my carb intake, so it's hard to get my usual reps with my maximum lifts. Even then, though, it's only two days out of that week, as I'll train Monday and Tuesday before resting the three days prior to Saturday showtime.

Forget about just being big at all costs, with no thought to the other attributes of a great bodybuilder. That's not the secret to winning, or even to just looking good. Being big doesn't mean you'll appear big onstage. If you want to win, you have to get cut, and pay attention to all the details that go into displaying the complete package.

ON EGO LIFTING...

I see all these guys in the gym lifting more than me. What am I doing wrong?

An inspection of pro bodybuilders might leave you with the impression that our ultimate goal is to attain a perfect physique or lift some specific amount of weight. Nothing could be further from the truth; in fact, everything's wrong with that seemingly innocent notion.

No thoughtful athlete in this sport is motivated by ego or greed, because neither of those properties has the strength to withstand the sacrifice inherent in what we do. Bodybuilding has no finish line. It's a way of life, driven by the concept of infinite ability to improve.

My suggestion is to forget about increasing your lifts to match what you see other people doing, and concentrate instead on putting everything you can into each workout. As your totality of strength and form improves, your poundages will increase as well, and at a faster rate than if you concentrate on moving more in each specific exercise.

Pushing yourself too hard, or working to match someone else, is a blueprint for failure. In bodybuilding, the best and only true gauge of progress is measurement against yourself. As long as you continually improve, it doesn't matter what people are doing around you. Control what you can, and if you're lifting less than the guy on the bench press next to you, so what? Trust me, if you stick to it and continually make incremental gains in your strength and your physique, you will soon be miles ahead of 90% of the other people at your gym. So many people get distracted by running some nonexistent race against others, or some ideal they think they must attain. Keep the focus on you, and give yourself kudos for the small victories you do accomplish along the way, whether it be a new pound of muscle this month or hoisting five more pounds on your deadlift this week vs. last. Stay on your path, and you'll get to the destination you seek in due time.

ON REP SCHEMES...

What's the ideal number of reps for maximal muscle growth?

Throughout this book, I've been preaching the 10–15 rep range that I use for most of my exercises. But let's take that notion of rep counting for a moment and put it to further scrutiny, because I would like to make an important point.

You can count reps all you want, but don't count on the act of counting for maximum growth. It's an oft-heard phrase, but it bears repeating here: Bodybuilding is about quality, not quantity.

Scientists will produce data proving one rep range, or number of total sets, or a training cycle, or any number of training variables is the one and best answer to the question of what is the best way to bodybuild. But I'll argue it's much simpler than all of that. It all comes down to the pump you're able to build within a muscle. That's the ultimate gauge of whether everything you're doing in your training is worthwhile.

People constantly comment on the amount of weight I use, my high reps and my basic exercises, saying they all can be improved upon in some way, but my choices are solely dictated by my quest for developing a specific sensation in the target muscle. I don't tackle a workout obsessed with being able to lift a specific number of pounds for a specific number of repetitions. My goal is to lift whatever it takes, for however many reps and sets it takes, to feel a good full pump in the muscle.

Finding that ideal combination of weight and reps for the optimum pump is a task that can't be taken casually. It demands extensive experimentation. The 10–15 rep rule of thumb is only a starting point — it may be far from ideal for your body. Maybe the ideal for you is six, or 12, but if you don't have a good pump after 15 reps, the weight is too light or you're cheating through your set. If you reach failure at three or six reps without building a pump, the weight is too heavy or you're not focusing on the muscle.

You'll probably find that the number of reps for building an ideal pump varies within each muscle group, according to the adjustments your body needs to make for balance and strength. Power-plane movements, such as squats, military presses, deadlifts and bench presses, have a higher

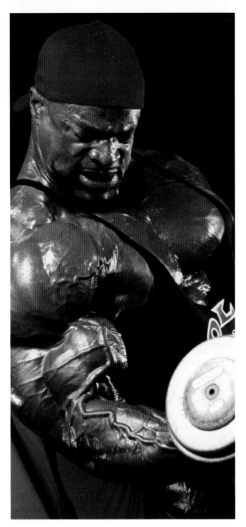

weight-per-rep ratio, so they usually require fewer reps to build a full pump. Exercises such as barbell curls, lateral raises or cable pressdowns have a lower weight-per-rep ratio, so they usually require higher reps to build a full pump. Even at that, other factors — your proportions, torso mass and relative length and strength of your arms and legs — can affect the number of reps you'll need.

If you want to experiment, try this scenario next time you're training. Start with a weight that builds a good pump at 12 reps, then concentrate harder to see if you can get an even better pump in 15 reps at the same weight. Progressively increase the weight over each set in an attempt to build the same or better pump with

fewer reps. If you begin to lose the pump, you've gone too far; stay at your best-pump combination until your strength signals that you're ready to increase the weight.

To end, a warning: Never be content merely copying the rep ranges of top pros, or even shooting for some number as the end of a set with no mind to the quality of those reps. Instead, think only of building a pump with smooth, firm reps and perfect control. That's the only way to achieve the growth you seek.

ON REP SPEED...

What's the optimal rep speed for building mass?

The speed, smoothness, consistency and control of reps vary according to the exercise, its purpose, the bodypart and the ordinal position of the set in your workout.

(1) THE EXERCISE: Repetition speed will vary, depending upon whether the exercise is performed with cables, free weights or a machine. The unique advantage of cables is that since resistance is even over the entire range of motion, you can concentrate on isolating a specific muscle to do the work and on maintaining a contraction of that muscle throughout the duration of the set. The most effective use of cables is by means of slower repetitions, with a pace that's consistent through both the contraction and extension phases.

With free weights, the moment of force, or resistance, varies through the arc of the movement: At some points, the weight feels heavier than at others, just the opposite of the sensation associated with cables. You have to apply more power at those higher resistance points than at others, which means you have to accelerate or decelerate your rep, or "cheat," in order to complete it. This "cheating"

brings into play ancillary muscles for added force, which reduces your ability to isolate the muscle, but amplifies the resistance against it, causing it to work harder, consequently increasing in mass. So free weights are more effectively employed by reps that are controlled but slightly more explosive.

Machines are a good middle ground between cables and free weights. They don't allow for as precise isolation as cable moves, but they do provide consistent resistance over the entire range of motion. At the same time, machines avoid the stabilizing and balancing distractions of free weights, and they allow you to apply the mass-building leverage of free weights. Reps that are slow and controlled during the extension and explosive during the contraction are most effective when using machines.

(2) THE PURPOSE: Speed of repetition is also governed by whether the exercise you're doing is for defining and shaping an isolated muscle, or whether it's for building overall mass of the muscle group. If the former, your reps should be slightly slower, smoother, more consistent and more controlled. If the latter, they should be more explosive and, perhaps, faster.

(3) THE BODYPART: Smaller bodyparts require more isolated control than larger bodyparts, so reps for the exercises are usually slower and more consistent. However, there are times when you want to build an intense burn in a muscle and for that you should pump your reps relatively fast. For big bodyparts, such as chest, back and quads, you'll be using much more weight, so your reps will naturally be slower.

(4) THE ORDINAL POSITION OF THE SET: The speed of your reps will depend on whether you're doing your warm-up set, your first working set or your heaviest set. Control your reps and keep them slow at the start of your warm-up set, then increase the pace to work out the stiffness of the muscle group and pump it full of blood. Your first working set should be controlled and consistent, but at a slower pace, and your final heaviest set should be explosive on the contraction, and extra slow on the descent.

This brings us to the crux of the issue: When all is said and done, the speed of your reps is governed not by your will, but by the amount of weight you're lifting. If your goal is to reach failure at eight reps, you have no say regarding how fast those reps are performed. Pound them out as hard as you can to just barely make it all the way through the set with not a rep to spare. Obviously, the weight will cause your rep speed to decelerate as you proceed through the set, and your last rep may seem as though it's taking forever (you may be pushing as hard as you can, in other words explosively, but the bar may still be moving slowly).

Fast slow, moderate — none of those are as important as concentrating on keeping each rep tight through the entire range of motion and applying power smoothly and steadily during the contraction. Do the same with resistance during the extension and, on your last rep, give it everything you have. That's the secret to rep speed.

ON STRIATIONS...

How do I get those striations in my muscle?

You can't have striations without a proper diet, but don't think for a moment that training is less important. Both are needed to make sure layers of fat don't obscure your muscles and that individual muscles are sufficiently developed to stand out in distinct relief from one another.

In the pursuit of striations, I empha-

size these training tricks. From my years of experience, I've discovered that the following factors constitute the formula that will produce the highest quality of striated muscle in the shortest time.

(1) HEAVY WEIGHT: Striations don't come from surface muscularity, but from deep, thick, full and complete development of individual muscles, and the only way to achieve that is to train heavy enough to activate all of that muscle's fibers, from deep in its belly to its outermost tie-ins. That means stressing them from inside out with maximum weight resistance,

forcing them to pull and strain to stretch their capacity. Try for heavier lifts every workout.

(2) 10-15 REPS PER SET: Individual muscles must be worked to their capacity for every set, and the most efficient means I've found to achieve that state is with a minimum of 10 reps per set — and often as many as 15. Commanding and individual muscle to perform the bulk of the work from the very first repetition of a set is easy when you're using light weight, but not enough stress is applied. The first few reps with heavy weight, however, require you to concentrate more on

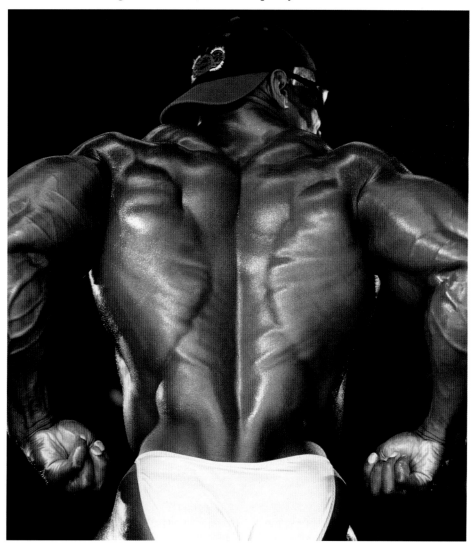

overcoming and controlling the resistance than on the specific muscle's contractions and extensions. Not until the fourth or fifth rep does a muscle adjust to flexing that heavy weight solely by itself to reach optimum efficiency. By aiming for higher reps, I'm using those first few reps to acquaint the muscle with the weight. Thereafter, I'm getting 5–10 perfect heavy contractions and extensions before the set is finished.

(3) SUPERSETS, TRI-SETS & GIANT SETS: The best technique I've found for pumping a muscle up to maximum blood volume is with supersets, tri-sets or giant sets. With the proper amount of control and weight, you can — with one set — build almost perfect blood volume in a specific muscle, pressing it out through its fibers to give it distinctive striations, but additional super, tri- or giant sets virtually guarantee this effect. Furthermore, they sustain that maximum blood volume longer than a single set does. (A superset is two exercises done back to back with no rest in between; a tri-set is three exercises; and a giant set is four or more.)

(4) COMPLETE RANGE OF MOTION: The easiest way to feel how a muscle is performing is to use a full range of motion, smoothly extending all the way, then contracting likewise, intensifying the squeeze as you go. This allows you to mentally become one with that muscle, almost as if you're commanding it to pop out separately from its adjacent fibers.

(5) VISUALIZE STRIATIONS: If you see them in your mind's eye, they'll come. With every extension and contraction, concentrate on individual fibers becoming more massive, apart from all the others. Think bigger, and your muscles will become bigger and more visibly separated.

Remember that your body is the sum of all of its parts, and striation training is focusing on each individual part.

ON GETTING THAT "HARD" LOOK...

What kind of workout regimen should I do to get that cut, hard look pros have onstage?

Pinning all of your hardness hopes on a specific workout regimen is futile. First of all, obsessing about reps, sets and poundages tempts you to forget about your dietary responsibilities. Secondly, those numbers by themselves have little to do with either muscle or cuts. If your major concern is to rep away bodyfat, you'll rep away a substantial amount of muscle mass with it. Even a preoccupation with lifting heavy weights has its pitfall, forcing you to forego proper muscle-building techniques in favor of strength. That's what breeds those huge puffy guys I see in the gym every day, the ones who throw around monster weight without getting anything out of it. They're bulky, but not what I consider big — and they never come close to being hard.

Here's the simple truth: I have that hard look not because I possess some kind of encyclopedic knowledge of diet foods, and not because I've figured out the "perfect" number of exercises, sets and poundages. I have that look because I train deep. That means I not only want to feel the exercise penetrating into its targeted muscle, but also into every other muscle that helps stabilize and support it. Ideally, I'd like every set to build a burn throughout my entire body. The deeper the burn, the harder your muscularity. Why else do you think I do so many free-weight compound-movement exercises with extremely heavy weight?

I do them to tear down a larger volume of muscle fibers, so an even larger volume will grow out of the rubble.

Now, how do I get those reps to penetrate so deep? Hyper-isolated movements and light weight don't work. That's like using a nail when you should be using a railroad spike: you'll barely penetrate the surface. Low reps are also insufficient, like hammering a railroad spike only halfway to its hilt. Instead, I pound at every rep with all the power and fury I can muster, as if that railroad spike has all the resistance of a fence post. Rep after rep, I hammer it with blistering intensity, until it hits bottom and sends shock waves scattering to the farthest corners of my body. That's training deep.

Compound movements, heavy weight and relentless reps: You need all three for hardness, and they translate into your workout as follows. For every bodypart, you need at least one barbell exercise and one dumbbell exercise. Two of each is even better. Do four sets of every exercise. Put on whatever weight limits you to 10 reps, then do 12. Next time, make it 15.

Make sure the weight is heavy enough so that your very first rep pulls at your muscle and starts the pump. By the time you reach your 12th rep, you should feel every muscle in the region burning and tugging, straining in the opposite direction to help the assaulted bodypart defend itself against total annihilation.

Even at that point, I never let up. That's when I go to my next exercise and drive that burn in from a different direction — heavier, harder, with more reps; maybe with supersets or giant sets, maybe even finishing with a powerlifting movement heavier than my first exercise, or with something crazy, such as parking-lot lunges.

Mine is a lonely existence, because no training partner can stay with me. But that also means I get to stand alone at the top of Mount Olympia.

ON INTENSITY...

Is there a technique I can use to increase my intensity? Or does it come naturally with experience?

I've always been very motivated, but not by the same goals often cited by others. There seems to be no shortage of advice for how to set goals. The so-called experts all parrot each other with the chorus that to motivate yourself, all you have to do is be very clear about what your long-term goals are, then set achievable short-term goals to get there. In my opinion, that's living in a dream world. They're thinking only of that blissful, trouble-free destination and ignoring the hard road to get there.

I'm just the opposite. I like to think of my goal not as the destination, but as the long, hard, rocky road of sacrifice along which I have to claw my way. That's what makes me proud, that's what makes me burn with even more intensity the next time I face a workout: The challenge of fighting the fight.

How does this philosophy sustain my intensity through all aspects of my life? Again, it's the opposite of what you usually hear. I don't visualize myself standing onstage with the best physique in the world, being showered with adoration. Instead, I humble myself with reality. I think of the fact that I have to go to the gym in a couple of hours and place myself under a weight I've never been able to lift, or do that one additional rep I've never been able to get.

I've also never bought into the notion that a few hard sets are all that a bodybuilder should do on a given day. Again, it's just the opposite. Push yourself to a physical extreme so that you can enter a region that is governed by simple reflexes. Only there can you find your "zone," where all muscle groups in your body function in their most natural and efficient manner.

I know how hard it is to stay focused on training from one week to the next. I have the Mr. O contest to keep me motivated, but for the average bodybuilder, the payback is far less concrete. In the end, it's a mental challenge to become successful, whether you're competing or not. Just remember, you can't accomplish anything with the workouts in this book unless you put your mind to work for your body every time you train.

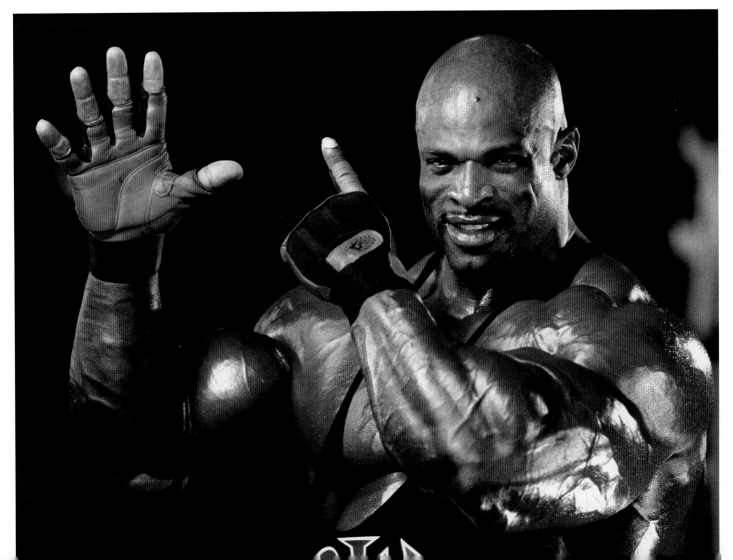

RONNIE'S OLYMPIA WINS

Some champions seemed destined for greatness. From the very beginning of their career, you see hints that one day, they could very well become the best in their sport. In bodybuilding, perhaps it's one-in-a-million genetic structure, or standout bodyparts that set a new standard in development, or a charisma to own any stage they step on combined with a killer instinct that leads them to crush the competition.

In 1998, Ken "Flex" Wheeler was that champion. After six-time victor Dorian Yates' retirement, bodybuilding pundits the world over thought that it was finally the moment for Wheeler. After all, from the very start of his pro career in 1993, when he won four shows (including the Arnold Classic) and finished second in two others (including the Mr. Olympia), it seemed it was only a matter of time until the gifted athlete with the classic lines and almost flawless physique earned a Sandow.

As they say in sports, "That's why we play the games." Because, instead of the 1998 Mr. Olympia becoming Wheeler's crowning achievement, it became the first step in an improbable and incredible run at the history books. That year, a man who finished ninth in 1997 would enter the limelight and score a stunning upset.

He would go on to prove it was no fluke, and now stands as arguably the greatest bodybuilder who ever lived: Ronnie Coleman, now an eight-time winner of his profession's most coveted and celebrated title, tied with his idol Lee Haney for that prestigious honor. Here, in the words of *Flex* magazine's group editorial director Peter McGough, is Coleman's journey to immortality.

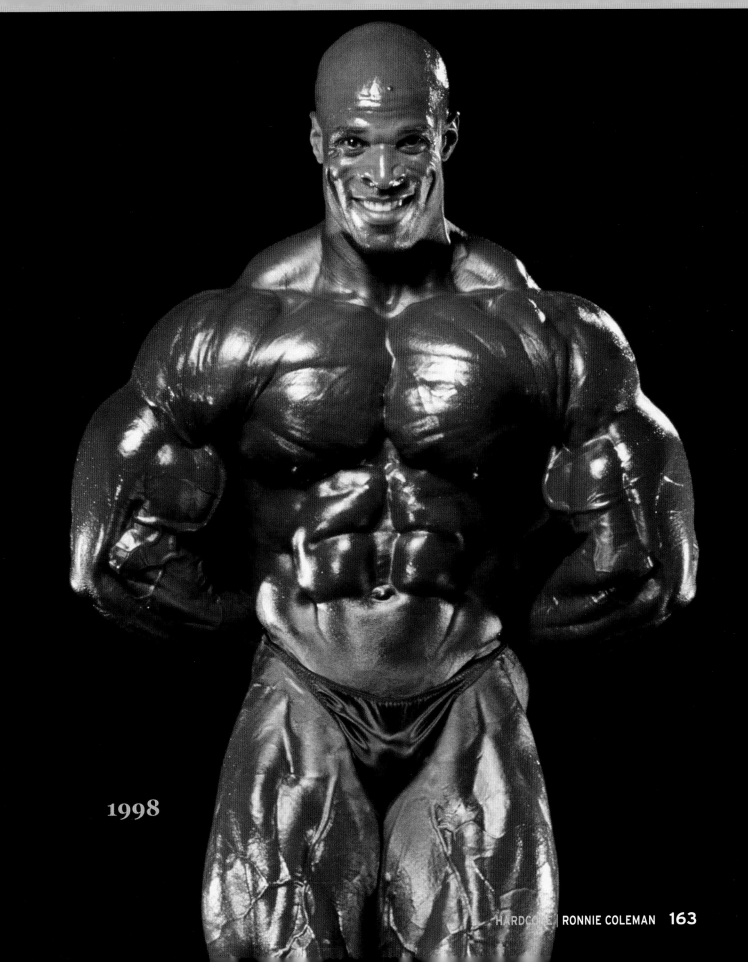

1998

1998 MR. OLYMPIA

October 10, 1998: Madison Square Garden, New York

With the retirement of Dorian Yates, the red-hot favorite for the 1998 Mr. Olympia was Flex Wheeler. Trouble was no one told 250-pound Ronnie Coleman, whose best Olympia placing had been sixth in 1996. As Coleman strode out at the start of proceedings, he was hard and cut and in his best shape ever. Although he was trailing Wheeler after the first two rounds, he finished like a locomotive at full speed to take the final two rounds. As he was announced " Mr. Olympia," 5,000 fans erupted into celebration, Coleman dropped to the floor sobbing uncontrollably and a dynasty was born.
Top Ten: 10) Jean-Pierre Fux; 9) Mike Matarazzo; 8) Ernie Taylor; 7) Lee Priest; 6) Chris Cormier; 5) Shawn Ray; 4) Kevin Levrone; 3) Nasser El Sonbaty; 2) Flex Wheeler; 1) Ronnie Coleman.

1999 MR. OLYMPIA

October 23, 1999: Mandalay Bay Resort & Casino, Las Vegas

In the glitzy locale of Las Vegas, a larger than life city perfect for showcasing larger than life bodybuilders, a 257-pound Ronnie Coleman outmuscled 15 other contenders as he steam-rolled his way to unanimous victory in his first defense of the Mr. Olympia crown. Commenting after his victory, he said, "I knew what it took to win this title in the first place, so I knew what it would take to repeat. Why change what works. I looked exactly like I wanted to look. All my goals were achieved.

And yes, I'm much more confident than I used to be because .... I'm Mr. Olympia, baby!"
Top Ten: 10) Milos Sarcev; 9) Dexter Jackson; 8) Lee Priest; 7) Paul Dillett; 6) Nasser El Sonbaty; 5) Shawn Ray; 4) Kevin Levrone; 3) Chris Cormier; 2) Flex Wheeler; 1) Ronnie Coleman.

2000 MR. OLYMPIA

October 21, 2000: Mandalay Bay Resort & Casino, Las Vegas

After being chased to the wire in the previous two years by Flex Wheeler, Coleman's main adversary this time out was Kevin Levrone, who gave the champ all the trouble he could handle. But at 264 pounds, Coleman was equal to the task and in this, his third Olympia victory, it was clear he had built a psychological advantage over his rivals. This was in equal part deference to Coleman being a multiple Mr. Olympia winner and not a one-hit wonder, and also his own level of confidence that had now reached charismatic levels.
Top Ten: 10) Orville Burke; 9) Dexter Jackson; 8) Jay Cutler; 7) Markus Rühl; 6) Lee Priest; 5) Nasser El Sonbaty; 4) Shawn Ray; 3) Flex Wheeler; 2) Kevin Levrone; 1) Ronnie Coleman.

2001 MR. OLYMPIA

October 27, 2001: Mandalay Bay Resort & Casino, Las Vegas

In this post 9/11 Olympia, patriotism was the star attraction as competitors and audience alike united to celebrate the sport they loved. That being said, this was the most controversial victory of Coleman's reign. Jay Cutler nearly

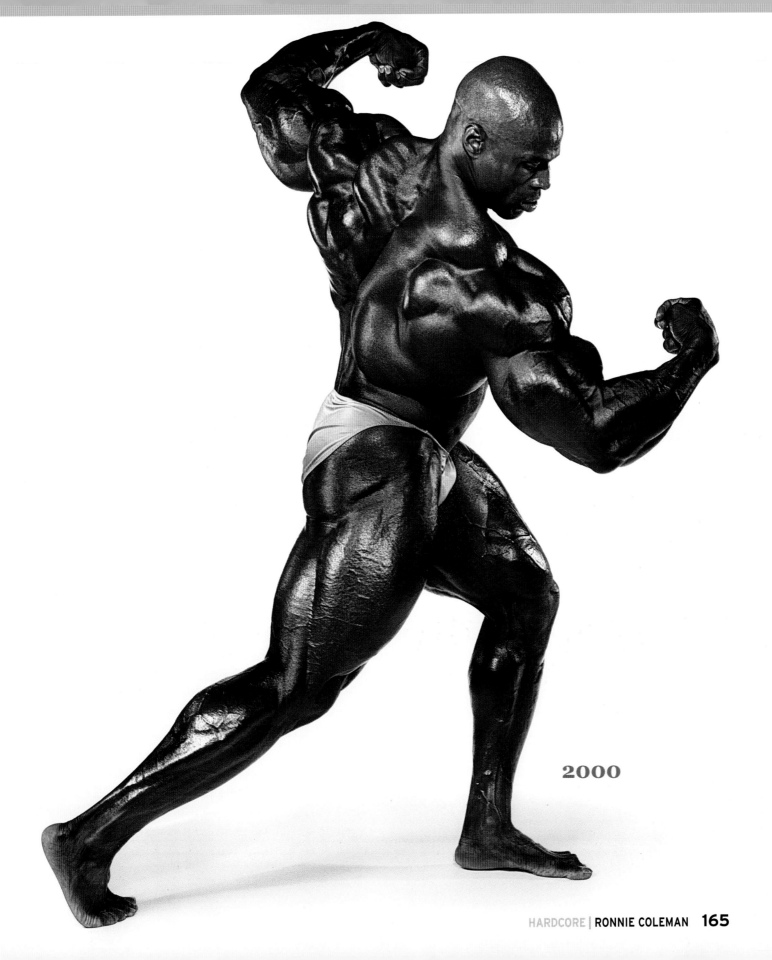

2000

spoiled Ronnie's Olympia party as he took the lead after the first two rounds of prejudging. Like a true champ, the 265-pound Coleman seemed unphased as in an interlude befitting of the general spirit of the weekend, he posed in a pair of stars and stripes trunks. Eventually he clawed his way back into contention during the evening and went ahead after the final posedown round, and was thus for the fourth time announced Mr. Olympia. For the fourth time, he hit the deck afterward, as the emotion of the moment overwhelmed him.

Top Ten: 10) King Kamali; 9) Nasser El Sonbaty; 8) Dexter Jackson; 7) Dennis James; 6) Orville Burke; 5) Chris Cormier; 4) Shawn Ray; 3) Kevin Levrone; 2) Jay Cutler; 1) Ronnie Coleman.

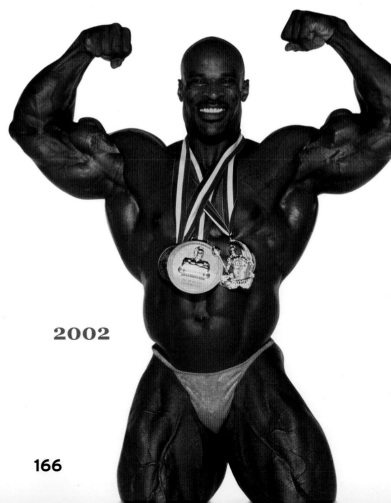

2002

2002 MR. OLYMPIA

October 19, 2002: Mandalay Bay Resort & Casino, Las Vegas

After running the champ close in 2001, Jay Cutler skipped this year's rendition but Coleman still hand his hands full with a resurgent Kevin Levrone, whose never-say-die attitude took this down to the wire. At 245 pounds, Ronnie was 20 pounds lighter than the previous year, and although Levrone held his own in the upper body department, the reigning Mr. Olympia's all round better leg development was the deciding factor. Post-morteming the result, the now five-time Mr. Olympia said: "I know what I'm here to do. God has put me here for a purpose, and I'm going to do His work, go wherever He leads me. I'm just happy to be here."

Top Ten: 10) Dennis James; 9) Orville Burke; 8) Markus Rühl; 7) Flex Wheeler; 6) Lee Priest; 5) Günter Schlierkamp; 4) Dexter Jackson; 3) Chris Cormier; 2) Kevin Levrone; 1) Ronnie Coleman.

2003 MR. OLYMPIA

October 25, 2003: Mandalay Bay Resort & Casino, Las Vegas

With joyful tears gushing down his cheeks, Ronnie Coleman, in addressing the Mandalay Bay crowd after his sixth win, said, "I got mad love for y'all." What he also had was an awesome 287-pound amalgam of muscle the likes of which had never been seen before. After two close runs in the previous two years (and criticisms that he had been much too light in 2002) Coleman put on 22 pounds and clinched this one hands down from the moment he first appeared onstage. This wasn't really a title defense it was a celebration of the ninth wonder of the world.

Top Ten: 10) Ernie Taylor; 9) Melvin Anthony; 8) Troy Alves; 7) Darrem Charles; 6) Kevin Levrone; 5) Günter Schlierkamp; 4) Dennis James; 3) Dexter Jackson; 2) Jay Cutler; 1) Ronnie Coleman.

2004 MR. OLYMPIA

October 30, 2004: Mandalay Bay Resort & Casino, Las Vegas

For this year's event star power (with Governor Arnold Schwarzenegger, Sylvester Stallone, Triple H and Tom Arnold in attendance) had never been bigger, and neither had Ronnie Coleman. At 296 pounds the champ eclipsed even the dimensions of the previous year and once again swept to a straight firsts victory with Jay Cutler – for the third time – being just a Ronnie Coleman away from a Sandow. Basking in his seventh heaven victory, Coleman remarked afterward, "The more I win the greater the feeling is. The ultimate goal is to beat Lee Haney's [eight titles] record. Right now I want to enjoy number seven and then get started going for number eight."

Top Ten: 10) Darrem Charles; 9) Victor Martinez; 8) Dennis James; 7) Chris Cormier; 6) Günter Schlierkamp; 5) Markus Rühl; 4) Dexter Jackson; 3) Gustavo Badell; 2) Jay Cutler; 1) Ronnie Coleman.

2005 MR. OLYMPIA

October 15, 2005: Orleans Arena, Las Vegas

In the new high-tech environs of the Orleans Arena, the buzz all year had been the IFBB's

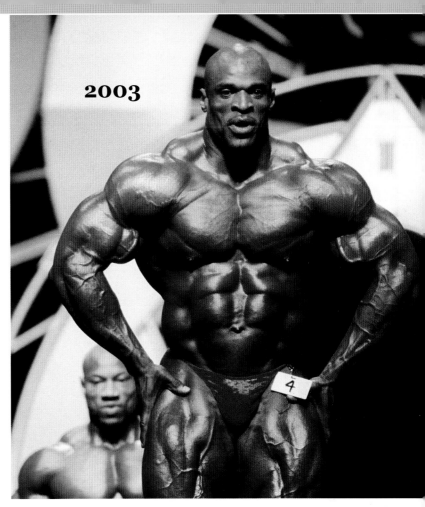

2003

edict to penalize any distension of the stomach. Proving he is a man for all seasons, Coleman trimmed down to 275 pounds and neutralized any chance that he would be dethroned by the new decree, and he again battled his way to the top spot. In a reflective mood he mused, "It's kind of unbelievable. I came into this thing in 1998, glad to win one, and now its eight later." He shook his head, almost in disbelief. "It's good to be king." And king he truly is, because in the history of bodybuilding nobody came from further back and ascended higher than Ronnie Coleman.

Top Ten: 10) Mustafa Mohammad; 9) Darrem Charles; 8) Branch Warren; 7) Melvin Anthony; 6) Dennis James; 5) Victor Martinez; 4) Günter Schlierkamp; 3) Gustavo Badell; 2) Jay Cutler; 1) Ronnie Coleman.

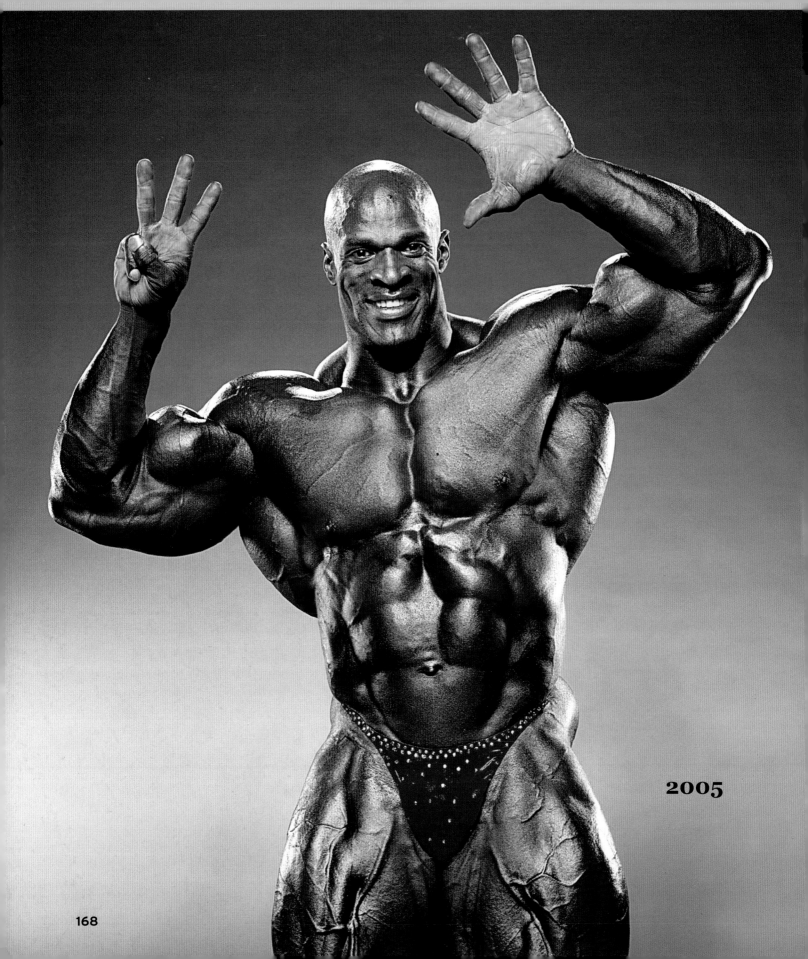

2005